Best of Five MCQs for MRCPsych Paper 1

Best of Five MCQs for MRCPsych Paper 1

Lena Palaniyappan
Academic Clinical Fellow, Institute of Neurosciences, Newcastle University and Specialty Registrar, Division of Psychiatry, Royal Victoria Infirmary, Newcastle, UK

Rajeev Krishnadas
Clinical Lecturer, Sackler Institute of Psychobiological Research, University of Glasgow, Glasgow, UK

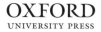

OXFORD
UNIVERSITY PRESS

OXFORD
UNIVERSITY PRESS

Great Clarendon Street, Oxford OX2 6DP

Oxford University Press is a department of the University of Oxford.
It furthers the University's objective of excellence in research, scholarship,
and education by publishing worldwide in

Oxford New York

Auckland Cape Town Dar es Salaam Hong Kong Karachi
Kuala Lumpur Madrid Melbourne Mexico City Nairobi
New Delhi Shanghai Taipei Toronto

With offices in

Argentina Austria Brazil Chile Czech Republic France Greece
Guatemala Hungary Italy Japan Poland Portugal Singapore
South Korea Switzerland Thailand Turkey Ukraine Vietnam

Oxford is a registered trade mark of Oxford University Press
in the UK and in certain other countries

Published in the United States
by Oxford University Press Inc., New York

© Oxford University Press, 2009

British Library Cataloguing in Publication Data
Data available

Library of Congress Cataloguing in Publication Data
Data available

Typeset by Cepha Imaging Private Ltd., Bangalore, India
Printed in the United Kingdom by CPI Antony Rowe

ISBN 978–0–19–955077–7

10 9 8 7 6 5 4 3 2

FOREWORD

I am delighted and honoured to be asked to write a foreword for this excellent book.

The authors are to be commended in producing an excellent series of relevant MCQ questions. These will form about 70% of Papers I to III in the revised MRCPsych examination. Many trainees have difficulties with this kind of question – particularly with the harder ones which will only increase in frequency as the examiners struggle to make up new questions with each diet! The MCQs in this volume have the characteristics of being both fair and stretching. Comprehensive and clear answers to these questions with references from easily available, standard text books are included. The whole of the prescribed MRCPsych syllabus has been covered in these questions and answers. The best answer to many questions like this is 'I'll look it up', but this is not a recourse that one can use in exams and this book should help considerably in passing them.

Professor Nicol Ferrier
Newcastle University

ACKNOWLEDGEMENT

This work began with an idea of a producing revision aids for new MRCPsych exams. A number of people helped us to conceive, nurture and develop this idea, and transform it to its current physical form.

We are thankful to all those who have taught us and supervised us over the years, imparting curiosity to learn, and to teach psychiatry.

Dr Thambirajah provided the much needed dopamine to our brains' reward areas! In addition he reviewed a few chapters in this series. We are deeply indebted to our other reviewers Dr David Christmas, Dr Niraj Ahuja and Dr Ranjit Krishnadas.

A special thanks to Prof Ferrier for writing the foreword.

Chris Reid, Jo Hardern & Fiona Goodgame from OUP deserve special mention for their patience and perseverance.

Heartfelt thanks to Priya and Sindhu; we could not have seen this book as it is now but for their sacrifice of many relaxing evenings and leisurely weekends!

CONTENTS

INTRODUCTION

THE MRCPSYCH PAPER 1:
TAKING THE BULL BY ITS HORNS

MRCPsych exams are the most important exams a psychiatry trainee in the UK will sit during his or her career. Passing the MRCPsych is the most visible of the criteria that demonstrate the achievement of a number of competencies during the training. Since spring 2008, there has been a significant change in the pattern of the exam. The structure, syllabus, and the format of questions have changed significantly.

WHO CAN SIT THE EXAM?

The details are clearly given in the Royal College website. They are summarized below for quick reference. Please note that these are subject to change and so we recommend checking with information at **www.rcpsych.ac.uk** before you apply.

Training requirements[1]
The college has brought out new exam regulations that are to come into effect from January 2009. Candidates must have completed the mandatory training period of 12 months of post foundation training in psychiatry by the date of sitting the written exams. Posts must be part of a programme of training approved by PMETB OR recognised by the Hospital or Trusts as having specific time, programme (journal clubs, grand rounds, teaching, supervision, etc.) and funds allocated for training. Individual posts can be of either 4 or 6 months duration. It could be a 12 month post in adult psychiatry OR a 6 month post in old age psychiatry and a 6 month post of adult psychiatry OR a combination of 4 month posts in adult or old age psychiatry but with a minimum of 6 months in adult psychiatry.

Although the college has taken out the time limit beyond 12 months up to when a person can take the exam, they still recommend certain time frames when these exams can be taken ideally. For paper 1, it is 12-18 months, for paper 2, 18-24 months and for paper 3, it is 18-30 months. Paper 1 and 2 are passed permanently, but the results of paper 3 can be banked only for 635 days. Because the practical exam (CASC) can be sat only after 30 months (even if you pass all the theory exams in 12 months), it would make sense to delay taking the paper 3 after fulfilling the 30 month requirement for CASC. A person can sit the written exam any number of times.

In addition to the above, there are Work place based assessment (WPBA), Annual review of competency progression (ARCP) assessment and sponsorship requirements that have to be fulfilled as part of the training requirement.

WHAT IS PAPER I?

The MRCPsych Paper I is 3 hours long and contains 200 questions. The paper consists of multiple choice questions (MCQ, 75%) and extended matching items (EMI, 25%).

MCQs are in the 'best of five' (BOF) format. This type of MCQ comprises a question stem of varying length, followed by a list of five options. Candidates should choose the single best option that fits the question stem.

The college has retained the EMI format from the previous pattern in the new format. In the EMIs candidates are initially orientated by being given a theme for each set of EMIs, followed by a lead-in statement explaining what the candidate is being asked to do. This is followed by an option list, set out in a logical order. Finally, the vignettes are given and the candidate is asked to choose one or more best options from the option list.

One mark is given for each correct answer in both MCQs and EMIs. Candidates are advised to attempt all questions. No marks are deducted for incorrect answers.

Topics/syllabus for the Paper I exam

A rough guideline to the syllabus and distribution of questions, as given by the college, is shown in Table 1. The college gives a detailed curriculum of what is expected to be known in each topic, but how much is necessary for Paper I has not been specified. Please refer to **www.rcpsych.ac.uk** for any changes (which are inevitable with any evolving exam).

HOW TO PREPARE FOR THE EXAM

Preparation for the exam starts the very day the training starts. This should be directed towards gaining the requirements towards sitting the exam, as well as getting a good knowledge of the theories that underlie the principles and practice of psychiatry.

Reading should ideally start on the very first day. It is best to start reading around the cases that a trainee sees on a daily basis at the outpatient clinics and inpatient unit. These cases could be discussed with the supervisor and used for case-based discussions. A good place would be to start with descriptive phenomenology. For example, discuss delusions seen in a patient during a supervision session. In the process, read around delusions from a standard textbook on psychopathology and discuss the different kinds of delusion, the formation of delusion, and differential diagnosis. So by the end of 10 months, the trainee would have covered most of core psychiatry, phenomenology, and psychopharmacology. It will be a good idea to get the timetable and the topics at the local deanery MRCPsych course and read the relevant material before going in for the teaching session. This is particularly relevant for psychology (where we may not get a lot of opportunity to discuss topics with a psychologist).

Table 1 The syllabus and distribution of questions for Paper I[2]

Content	No. of Questions
History and Mental State	12
Descriptive Psychopathology	24
Cognitive Assessment	10
Neurological Examination	10
Assessment	16
Description and Measurement	6
Diagnosis	12
Classification	8
Aetiology	12
Prevention of Psychological Disorder	6
Basic Psychopharmacology	14
Human Psychological Development	8
Social Psychology	4
Basic Psychological Processes	14
Dynamic Psychopathology	12
Basic Psychological Treatments	8
History of Psychiatry	8

At least 2 to 3 months leading up to the exam should be left for revision. It would be best to create a timetable with the syllabus and curriculum in mind so as not to leave out important topics. Reading during this period should be exam oriented and should be done along with practice multiple choice questions. This could be done on your own or in a study group. Preparing in a group helps to get an idea of where one stands with respect to the knowledge base.

Practice tests

It is best to take a number of mock and practice tests before the exam as these will give a fairly good idea of one's strengths and weaknesses. Unfortunately, since the exam formats have changed recently, it is difficult to get an idea of the college question banks and typical college favourites. A number of privately run revision courses give an opportunity to take mock examinations. It is best not to rely on these courses to learn a lot of theory at the last moment. These courses and materials should only be used to aid revision. But it is best to revise from material the candidate has already read once through the previous 10 months, rather than starting afresh. When selecting a course, it would make sense to choose one that offers a number of mock tests. If not, you could ask your local MRCPsych organizers to set up mock examinations as part of the course. It is best to do mock exams in the same paper and pencil format, using 200 questions; and timing it at 160 minutes.

Books to read

Knowledge does not come from textbooks alone. All kinds of resources are useful, including the internet, but it is best to base the core reading on standard textbooks. These textbooks should form the basis of reading, but reading should not be restricted to these.

The two reference books that we recommend are *Kaplan and Sadock's Synopsis of Psychiatry* (this is an American book, which is comprehensive, with DSM and ICD criteria, and forms excellent reading in psychology and psychopharmacology in addition to basic psychiatry) and the *New Oxford Textbook of Psychiatry*. Both are two volume textbooks.

As for core reading, the *Shorter Oxford Textbook of Psychiatry* is a very good text to begin with. Each chapter is written in an authoritative style and relevant to training in the UK. At the end of each section or topic there is a reference for further reading in the topic, which is invaluable.

Descriptive phenomenology forms the basis of diagnosis in psychiatry. There are two books that give a good account of descriptive phenomenology: *Fish's Clinical Psychopathology: Signs and Symptoms in Psychiatry* by Patricia Casey and *Symptoms in the Mind: An Introduction to Descriptive Psychopathology* by Andrew Sims, and revised recently by Femi Oyebode.

A good introductory textbook for psychopharmacology is Stephen Stahl's *Essential Psychopharmacology: Neuroscientific Basis and Practical Applications*. It is very lucid to read with a number of diagrams which help understanding of the basis of psychopharmacology. The book is also good for Papers 2 and 3.

There are a number of books for basic psychology: *Psychology: Themes and Variations* by Wayne Weiten is especially recommended. It is an American book which is very easy to read with a lot of examples. Thambirajah's *Psychological Basis of Psychiatry* is also a good book, specifically designed for MRCPsych exams.

Paper 1 MRCPsych revision techniques in summary
1. Avoid studying irrelevant details in books and other texts; as they are not tailor-made for the exam.
2. As there is no existing bank of 1000 or 1500 questions to revise and attempt the exam confidently, one should get the basic concepts straight and correct, in order to tackle any surprises.
3. Group study helps in many ways; but make sure your peers are motivated to fully participate in the groups. Nothing can be more unfruitful than three people getting together but studying in isolation.

4. Plan, plan, and plan! Structure your time according to the syllabus you have to revise. Spend equal time reading theory from books and solving BOFs.
5. There is no harm in utilizing all available materials before you attempt your exam – ask your senior ST trainees or colleagues and seek resources from revision courses and local MRCPsych teaching lectures.

APPROACH TO MULTIPLE CHOICE QUESTIONS[3, 4]

The MRCPsych exam is more than reading and understanding the core subject. It has also to do with the technique of attempting best of five MCQs. Unlike the old-style ISQ, the new style is a bit more difficult to do because the chance of getting the answer wrong is 80% compared to 50% with the older style. The very concept of selecting the best answer lies in the fact that there may be more than one right answer, but we need to choose the best answer. In order to do this you get 180 minutes to answer 200 questions that is less than 1 minute to answer a question. This means that the more familiar you are with the concepts, the faster you can answer and you will be able to spend more time on the more difficult and longer questions. It is said that in most medical examinations, candidates who answer half the questions correctly would score around the 50th or 60th percentile. A score of 65% (130/200) would place the examinee above the 80th percentile, whereas a score of 30% (30/200) would rank him or her below the 15th percentile.

Test performance will always be influenced by your test taking skills. Considering various test taking strategies and developing and perfecting them well in advance of the test date can help you concentrate better on the test itself. We recommend you try various techniques to find what works best for you. It should, in the end, help you to:
• increase your reading pace;
• focus on the most relevant information;
• eliminate as many options when you are not sure of the correct answer.
You require enough practice using the techniques so that it becomes second nature and you don't concentrate on anything but how to choose the correct answer when you actually sit the exam.

Timing
Time management is an important skill for exam success. As mentioned above, the test has 200 questions to be answered in 3 hours which leaves about 54 seconds per question. Each time you spend more than 54 seconds on a single question, time should be made up on other questions. Therefore it is essential to practise answering questions within a time limit to avoid pacing errors in the exam. This is where attempting a number of mock exams will help.

Approaching each question
There are several established techniques for tackling multiple choice questions which will help you to find the single best answer choice. One of these is classifying each question as easy, workable, or impossible. The basic aim in doing this is to
• answer all easy questions;
• figure out the answer to all the workable questions in a reasonable amount of time;
• make fast and intelligent guesses on the impossible ones.

Another technique is to read the answer choices first along with the last sentence of the question before reading through the question quickly, so as to extract the most relevant information as well as to consider each of the answer possibilities in the context of the question. This is especially relevant when the question stem is large, for example a case scenario.

Elimination is one of the best tools that can be used in a single best answer multiple choice exam. Excluding the possibility of one answer choice proportionately increases the probability of you choosing the right answer.

Since this is a paper and pencil exam, it is better to answer the questions in order, one by one; this reduces chances of skipping and accidentally marking the wrong question or skipping an item. To avoid these 'frame-shift' errors, answer difficult questions with your best guess, mark them for review, move on and come back to them if you have time at the end.

Random guessing
- There are no negative marks for wrong answers, so no question should be left unanswered.
- A hunch is probably better than a random guess; we also suggest selecting a choice which you recognize over another which is totally unfamiliar to you.
- It is never beneficial to pick random choices unless you are grossly out of time and not answering all the questions, in which case the best bet would be to select a single letter like 'C' and marking the remaining questions with it. It is obvious that in this case the chance of picking the correct answer decreases with more answer choices. It is also believed that MCQ makers prefer to hide the answers either in C or D, the middle-most choices, more often than in the periphery.
- It is also very important to not randomly guess the answers during your study and review sessions as well as the practice test sessions, as it may increase the tendency to do the same for the exam.
- As mentioned before, it is essential to take as many practice tests as possible to try the various techniques and select the ones that give you the best results.
- Use any extra time you might have to recheck your answers. Do not be casual in your review or you may overlook serious mistakes.
- Never give up. If you begin to feel frustrated try taking a 30 second breather. Remember your goals and keep in mind the effort and time you have spent in preparing for the exam compared with the small additional effort you will need to keep your focus and concentration throughout the exam.

Other things to do before the exam
Make arrangements for study leaves as early as possible. It is also important to find out how much private study leave you are entitled to. Make all the necessary swaps on the on call rota. Some deaneries arrange for stay and transport for the exam if there are a number of candidates taking the exam. Application forms should be sent well in time. If there are queries regarding applications, they should be clarified from the college at the earliest.

The day prior to exam, choose a good place to stay near the centre, even if it is expensive. As usual, it is important to get a good night's sleep. A good preparation should make you feel confident.

BOF MCQ exam techniques in summary
1. People who fail in new format exams do so not because they don't know the answer for some questions; it is because they think they know the answer and keep thinking about one question for 5 minutes or so, losing the remaining answers.
2. All questions carry one mark only, no matter how easy or difficult each one is. So why spend all your time on 'difficult ones'?
3. In the large, clinical vignette type of questions you may have many irrelevant details; at the same time you may also have valuable clues to solve the BOF. It is useful to read the last sentence, that is the question, quickly before reading large vignettes fully.
4. People have different styles of approaching BOF. Exclusion technique needs more time than direct answer picking; if your style is one of exclusion, make sure you practise well enough to carry this out faster during the exam.

AFTER THE EXAM

If you have some stamina left at the end of this huge ordeal, it is not a bad idea to start recollecting the questions to form a question bank which will be useful for future candidates. It is best to recollect the questions in the company of a couple of colleagues. It will be a good idea to get the questions back to the college tutor and this will help to arrange further teaching. This will also help you to prepare for Papers 2 and 3 in future.

READING LIST

General Psychiatry
Sadock BJ and Sadock VA. *Kaplan and Sadock's Synopsis of Psychiatry: Behavioral Sciences/Clinical Psychiatry*, 10th edn. Lippincott Williams and Wilkins, 2007.
Gelder MG *et al.*, eds. *New Oxford Textbook of Psychiatry*. Oxford University Press, 2000.
Gelder MG *et al.*, eds. *Shorter Oxford Textbook of Psychiatry*, 5th edn. Oxford University Press, 2006.

Psychopathology
Casey P and Kelly B. *Fish's Clinical Psychopathology: Signs and Symptoms in Psychiatry*. Gaskell, 2007.
Oyebode F. *Sims' Symptoms in the Mind: An Introduction to Descriptive Psychopathology*, 4th edn. UK: Elsevier Health Sciences, 2008.

Psychopharmacology
Stahl SM. *Essential Psychopharmacology: Neuroscientific Basis and Practical Application*, 3rd edn. Cambridge University Press, 2008.

Psychology
Weiten W. *Psychology: Themes and Variations*, 3rd edn. Brooks/Cole, 1995.
Thambirajah MS. *Psychological Basis of Psychiatry*. Elsevier, 2005.

History of psychiatry and psychiatric ethics
These topics are not fully covered in most textbooks. It may be useful to seek these topics from revision courses or local MRCPsych teachers. A visit to your local library for the reference books mentioned above may be useful too.

Wishing you all the best with the exams. Yes. Take the bull by its horns now!

[1] http://rcpsych.ac.uk/PDF/Exams%20Eligibility%20July%202008.pdf
[2] http://rcpsych.ac.uk/exams/about/mrcpsychpaperii.aspx
[3] Bhushan V, Le T. First Aid for the USMLE Step 1 (First Aid) (Paperback) McGraw Hill Higher Education; 16Rev Ed edition (1 Jan 2006)
[4] Princeton Review, Stein M, Hwang G. Cracking the Boards: USMLE Step 1, 3rd Edition (Princeton Review Series) (Paperback) Princeton Review; 3 edition (Dec 2000)

1. **Which of the following is NOT a facilitative message?**
   A. 'Run on' question
   B. Self disclosure
   C. 'I want' message
   D. Silence
   E. Interpretation

2. **A psychiatrist at an early stage of his initial assessment interview asks the patient, 'Can you tell me about your depression?' Which of the following interview techniques is he utilizing?**
   A. Closed-ended questions
   B. Open-ended questions
   C. Reflecting
   D. Facilitation
   E. Put down question

3. **Which of the following is an open-ended question?**
   A. Tell me about yourself?
   B. Could you tell me the name of the prime minister?
   C. It seems as if you feel people are against you?
   D. What do you find stressful in your job?
   E. Do you have trouble falling asleep?

4. **During a clinical interview the following statement is made by the clinician: 'So you have been anxious since these changes occurred at your work place.' Which of the following interview technique best describes the above statement?**
   A. Facilitation
   B. Open-ended question
   C. Closed-ended question
   D. Interpretation
   E. Reflecting

5. **Which of the following interview techniques is least directive?**

    A. Limit setting
    B. Summarizing
    C. Re-direction
    D. Repetitive questioning
    E. Narrow-focused questions

6. **Which of the following is a supportive intervention during a clinical interview process?**

    A. Open-ended questions
    B. Acknowledgement of affect
    C. Confrontation
    D. Taking a medical history
    E. Summarization

7. **Which of the following statements is true when enquiring about suicidal ideation?**

    A. This should not be asked unless the patient volunteers information
    B. Asking about suicidal ideation can instil suicidal ideas in a person
    C. A person who intends to attempt suicide will never divulge
    D. Passive suicidal ideas must be enquired further for any plans made
    E. The aim of the assessment is to corner the patient into a disclosure

8. **'Do you ever hear voices commenting on what you are doing?' This question is usually asked to ascertain the presence of which one of the following?**

    A. Bleuler's primary symptoms
    B. Schneider's first-rank symptoms
    C. Command hallucinations
    D. Catatonic symptoms of schizophrenia
    E. Negative symptoms of schizophrenia

9. **Regarding the Mini Mental State Examination (MMSE), which of the following statements is true?**

    A. The subject is asked to guess the answer if unsure
    B. If a person scores 3 on serial sevens, and scores 4 on spelling WORLD backwards then the score for attention is 3
    C. On the reading test one point is scored if the patient reads 'Close your eyes' out loud
    D. Education affects the rate of change of scores in normal and dementia subjects
    E. MMSE scores are not affected by socioeconomic status of a subject

10. **Assessment of insight is an integral part of mental state examination in psychiatric practice. Regarding insight, which of the following statements is true?**
    A. Patients with schizophrenia will never have insight into their illness
    B. OCD being a neurosis, insight is always intact
    C. Intellectual insight is present when patients' awareness and understanding of their symptoms lead to a change in behaviour
    D. Intellectual insight is the highest level of insight
    E. Loss of insight is similar to the concept of anosognosia in neurological illness

11. **A patient with schizophrenia vividly describes how Martians are 'reverse freezing' earth to produce global warming. He stops to ask what you think about this. Choose the best response.**
    A. This is a fantastic theory. But I want to know more about this. Tell me, have you ever seen these Martians?
    B. This seems possible but there is no proof for all this. Tell me, have you ever seen these Martians?
    C. This cannot be true. Martians do not exist. Tell me, have you ever seen these Martians?
    D. Tell me, have you ever seen these Martians?
    E. What I think is not so important. I want to know more about what you think of this. Tell me, have you ever seen these Martians?

12. **Which one of the following is NOT an advisable first response when a patient discloses past sexual abuse at a clinical encounter?**
    A. Postpone discussing the issue
    B. Ask if she wants to say anything more about this now
    C. Ask if she has ever disclosed this to anyone
    D. Ask if she sees a link between this and her current difficulties
    E. None of the above

13. **Closed questions are best avoided in which of the following scenarios?**
    A. A patient with suspected malingering
    B. A guarded patient not answering spontaneously
    C. A suggestible patient with learning difficulty
    D. A psychotic patient who is actively hallucinating
    E. All of the above

14. **Which of the following is the single best question to discern premorbid personality of a patient?**
    A. How would you describe yourself?
    B. How would your friends describe you?
    C. What were you like before you became unwell?
    D. If we had met 10 years ago, what sort of person would I be talking to?
    E. None of the above

15. **Which of the following is not a discriminating question to screen for harmful use of alcohol?**
    A. Have you ever attempted to cut down your drinking?
    B. Do you get annoyed when people talk about your drinking?
    C. Have you ever felt guilty for drinking excessively?
    D. Do you drink every evening?
    E. Do you need a drink as soon as you wake up?

16. **A patient looks dishevelled, with unkempt hair and dirty, unwashed clothes. Self neglect is commonly noted in all of the following EXCEPT**
    A. Alcoholism
    B. Chronic schizophrenia
    C. Depression
    D. Dementia
    E. Social phobia

17. **A 57-year-old lady with many previous hospitalizations is brought by police to casualty. She is wearing full make-up, green lipstick, shiny green nail polish, and green jewellery. She asks everyone at the admission unit to call her Ms Green. Which of the following diagnoses is most consistent with the above presentation?**
    A. Mania
    B. Depression
    C. Panic attacks
    D. Obsessive compulsive disorder
    E. Learning disability

18. **Which of the following domains of cognition is tested by administering Serial Sevens Test?**
    A. Short-term memory
    B. Attention
    C. Language
    D. Registration
    E. Recall

19. **A 33-year-old man attending an out-patient clinic turns towards his left and spits out, muttering unintelligibly. He does this act at least three times in half an hour and appears very guarded. This gesture is suggestive of which of the following?**
    A. Depression
    B. Suicidal thinking
    C. Low self esteem
    D. Responding to hallucination
    E. Acute confusion

20. **A depressed patient does not smile or laugh when a joke is shared by a fellow patient. She shows a defect in which of the following aspects of mental state examination?**
    A. Stability of affect
    B. Reactivity of affect
    C. Congruence of affect
    D. All of the above
    E. None of the above

21. **An elderly patient in a stroke ward laughs all of a sudden inappropriately, and within a few minutes becomes tearful and cries for no reason. She exhibits an abnormality in which of the following aspects of mental state examination?**
    A. Stability of affect
    B. Reactivity of affect
    C. Congruence of affect
    D. All of the above
    E. None of the above

22. **Which of the following is the major difference between mood and affect in mental state examination?**
    A. Mood is short-lived while affect is longer lasting
    B. Mood is objective while affect is subjective
    C. Affect is transient but difficult to interpret
    D. Affect is transient and self reported
    E. None of the above

23. **Nihilistic delusions will be congruent with which of the following findings of mental state examination?**
    A. Depression
    B. Mania
    C. Depersonalization
    D. Grandiose delusion
    E. None of the above

24. **When eliciting suicide risk, which of the following questions should be avoided if possible?**
    A. Do you have any plans to kill yourself?
    B. How are you feeling in your mood?
    C. Have you ever considered life is not worth living?
    D. Have you ever wanted to go to sleep and never wake up?
    E. None of the above

25. Which of the following is not a manifestation of hypothyroidism?

A. Hypothermia
B. Sparing of the posterior column sensations
C. Dementia
D. Cerebellar ataxia
E. Loss of deep tendon reflexes

26. Russell's sign is usually associated with which one of the following disorders?

A. Schizophrenia
B. Bipolar disorder
C. Bulimia nervosa
D. Panic disorder
E. Somatization disorder

27. On physical examination, you notice that a person with a history of substance misuse now has pilo-erection, dilated pupils, rhinorrhea, and he is yawning frequently. Withdrawal from which of the following substances can cause this presentation?

A. Cocaine
B. Opiate
C. Cannabis
D. Alcohol
E. Amphetamine

28. A 50-year-old patient was brought to the A and E department in a confused state. On physical examination he has nystagmus, ocular palsy, and ataxia. Which of the following parts of clinical assessment is likely to be most relevant to this presentation?

A. Past psychiatric history
B. Assessment of insight
C. Alcohol use history
D. Developmental history
E. Family history of dementia

29. An 18-year-old male, recently started on a medication, presents to the A and E department with slow, long-sustained, contorting, involuntary movements and postures involving proximal limb and axial muscles. Which of the following medications is most likely to cause the above presentation?

A. Propranolol
B. Diazepam
C. Risperidone
D. Procyclidine
E. Sertraline

30. **A 21-year-old female presented to the emergency department with complaints of recurrent attacks of severe dizziness, lasting for 10 to 20 minutes. On examination during the episode of dizziness, there was no evidence of nystagmus. Which one of the following is true?**

    A. Her symptoms may be associated with fear of going to places from where escape is impossible
    B. Deafness is usually present
    C. Vertigo without nystagmus is suggestive of central vertigo of brainstem origin
    D. Antihistaminic medications are likely to be effective in this case
    E. None of the above

31. **A sudden onset of chorea is least likely in which of the following conditions?**

    A. Hyperthyroidism
    B. Hypoparathyroidism
    C. Pregnancy
    D. Hypernatremia
    E. Huntington's disease

32. **Which of the following is NOT a feature of subacute combined degeneration of the spinal cord?**

    A. Loss of pain and touch
    B. Sensory ataxia
    C. Loss of bladder tone
    D. Hyper-reflexia
    E. Absence of reflexes

33. **Which of the following physical symptoms is seen in factitious disorder?**

    A. Unexplained bleeding
    B. Recurrent hypoglycaemia
    C. Grid iron abdomen
    D. Haemoptysis
    E. All of the above

34. **A man admitted to the psychiatric intensive care unit with a manic episode, received 10 mg of haloperidol intramuscularly as he had turned violent. He became unresponsive shortly afterwards. On examination, there is evidence of confusion, labile BP, hyperthermia, rigidity, and dysphagia. What is the most important differential diagnosis?**

    A. Acute dystonia
    B. Neuroleptic malignant syndrome
    C. Tardive dyskinesia
    D. Akathisia
    E. Parkinsonism

35. **Which of the following questionnaires is used to identify psychiatric 'caseness' in the general population**

   A. MMPI
   B. HDRS
   C. GHQ
   D. YMRS
   E. Repertory Grid

36. **Characteristic feature of Argyll Robertson pupil include all of the following EXCEPT**

   A. Light near dissociation
   B. Irregular pupil
   C. Miosis
   D. Iris atrophy
   E. Flynn phenomenon

37. **Thunderclap headache is highly suggestive of which one of the following?**

   A. Subarachnoid haemorrhage
   B. Migraine
   C. Cluster headache
   D. Temporal arteritis
   E. Tension headache

38. **Waddling gait is characteristic of which of the following neurological difficulties?**

   A. Proximal muscle weakness
   B. Hemiplegia
   C. Cerebellar lesions
   D. Sensory ataxia
   E. Astasia abasia

39. **A 59-year-old man has a small, spastic tongue with significant difficulty in pronouncing consonants. On neurological examination, he has a brisk jaw jerk. Which of the following is the most likely explanation for the above presentation?**

   A. Bulbar palsy
   B. Pseudobulbar palsy
   C. Myasthenia gravis
   D. Extrapyramidal dysarthria
   E. Dysphonia

40. **When mimicking the use of a screwdriver a patient rotates his arm at the shoulder but fixes his elbow. Which of the following could be diagnosed with the above presentation?**
   A. Ideational apraxia
   B. Ideomotor apraxia
   C. Limb kinetic apraxia
   D. Conduction apraxia
   E. Conceptual apraxia

41. **A patient is asked to prepare a sandwich in order to test her ability to perform a sequence of acts. This test is aimed at demonstrating which of the following?**
   A. Ideational apraxia
   B. Ideomotor apraxia
   C. Limb kinetic apraxia
   D. Conduction apraxia
   E. Conceptual apraxia

42. **Syndrome of isolated loss of auditory comprehension and repetition, without any abnormality of speech, naming, reading, or writing is suggestive of which of the following?**
   A. Pure word deafness
   B. Wernicke's aphasia
   C. Broca's aphasia
   D. Anomic aphasia
   E. Transcortical aphasia

43. **A well-educated solicitor develops a sudden cerebrovascular deficit which results in loss of ability to read or write, though he is able to speak reasonably well. The dysfunction produced by the ischaemia is called**
   A. Alexia with agraphia
   B. Alexia without agraphia
   C. Transcortical aphasias
   D. Global aphasia
   E. Wernicke's aphasia

44. **Which of the following is NOT a feature of upper motor neurone lesion?**
   A. Hyper-reflexia
   B. Hypertonia
   C. Loss of voluntary movement
   D. Normal muscle bulk
   E. Fasciculations

45. **A 65-year-old patient has been drinking nearly 80 units of alcohol a week for the last 13 years. He has numerous physical complications of alcohol use including cirrhosis and cerebellar degeneration. Which of the following is NOT a feature of cerebellar dysfunction?**
    A. Positive Romberg's sign
    B. Positive finger nose test
    C. Positive heel shin test
    D. Dysdiadochokinesia
    E. Pendular knee jerk

46. **In a road traffic accident, a 34-year-old man sustains crush injury of the spine. One half of his spinal cord is damaged severely at the level of the tenth thoracic vertebra. Which of the following is a feature of hemisection of the spinal cord?**
    A. Contralateral weakness
    B. Contralateral loss of pain sensation
    C. Contralateral loss of proprioception
    D. Ipsilateral loss of temperature sensation
    E. The sensory level is at the same level as the lesion (T_{10})

47. **A patient presents in an agitated state with increased sweating and tremors. On examination she has signs of Grave's disease. Which is the commonest sign noted in thyroid ophthalmopathy?**
    A. Lid lag
    B. Lid retraction
    C. Compressive optic neuropathy
    D. Diplopia
    E. Conjunctival congestion

48. **Headache associated with ipsilateral nasal congestion, rhinorrhea, lacrimation, redness of the eye is characteristic of which of the following?**
    A. Classical migraine
    B. Tension headache
    C. Cluster headache
    D. Headache secondary to depression
    E. Temporal arteritis

49. **Epilepsy associated with learning disability, shagreen patches, and ash leaf macules are seen in which of the following?**
    A. Epidermal nevus syndrome
    B. Tuberous sclerosis
    C. Neurofibromatosis
    D. Sturge–Weber syndrome
    E. Fabry's disease

50. **Parkinsonian features associated with downward gaze palsy and pseudobulbar dysarthria is characteristic of which of the following conditions?**
    A. Multisystem atrophy
    B. Idiopathic Parkinson's disease
    C. Drug-induced parkinsonism
    D. Progressive supranuclear palsy
    E. Corticobasal degeneration

51. **All of the following conditions that affect the trigeminal nerve present with significant sensory loss EXCEPT**
    A. Multiple sclerosis
    B. Trigeminal neuralgia
    C. Acoustic neuroma
    D. Meningioma
    E. Neurofibroma

52. **Which of the following is a cause of bilateral facial nerve palsy?**
    A. Systemic lupus erythematosus
    B. Sarcoidosis
    C. Guillain–Barré syndrome
    D. Wernicke–Korsakoff syndrome
    E. All of the above

53. **A patient known to have bipolar illness is on lithium. Which of the following will prompt you to check his lithium levels?**
    A. Delayed ankle jerk
    B. Rising serum creatinine
    C. Dysarthria
    D. Fine tremor
    E. Alopecia

54. **Which one of the following is a physical sign noted in anorexia nervosa?**
    A. Lanugo hair
    B. Grey hair
    C. Brown hair
    D. Alopecia areata
    E. Thickened, coarse hair

55. **Sleep spindles and K complexes on electroencephalogram (EEG) are seen in which of the following phase of sleep?**
    A. REM phase
    B. Stage 1 NREM phase
    C. Stage 2 NREM phase
    D. Stage 3 NREM phase
    E. Stage 4 NREM phase

56. **Electroencephalogram (EEG) is a commonly used diagnostic test. Which of the following statements regarding EEG is NOT correct?**

A. EEG signals are generated by the cerebral cortex

B. EEG depends on afferent inputs from subcortical structures, including the thalamus and brainstem reticular formation

C. Alpha rhythm and sleep spindles are produced by thalamic activity

D. Diagnostic EEG does not routinely record the activity of inferior temporal cortex

E. EEG changes are often very specific to a disease

57. **A 32-year-old school teacher is admitted for constipation and acute abdominal pain. She experiences visual and tactile hallucinations with intense anxiety. She develops motor weakness of her legs on administration of hypnotics and diclofenac. Which of the following laboratory tests is indicated?**

A. Serum lipid levels

B. Serum folate

C. Urine glucose

D. Urine porphyrins

E. Serum ceruloplasmin

58. **Which of the following is NOT helpful in differentiating pseudoseizures from true epileptic seizures?**

A. Asymmetric movements of limbs and side-to-side movement of the head during ictal activity

B. Raised postictal prolactin levels

C. Ictal EEG

D. Long-lasting seizures that wax and wane over time

E. Having an established diagnosis of epilepsy in the past

59. **Clozapine is strongly associated with fatal agranulocytosis. Which of the following is true regarding clozapine-induced agranulocytosis?**

A. The risk of agranulocytosis is greatest in the first year

B. Patients must have weekly blood tests throughout clozapine treatment

C. After a year blood tests can be discontinued

D. An amber report from the monitoring body indicates that clozapine should be stopped immediately

E. A red alert indicates that clozapine could be restarted in a patient who previously had an amber report

60. **Which one of the following statements regarding the dexamethasone suppression test is FALSE?**

A. Healthy subjects show cortisol suppression on dexamethasone administration

B. Depressed patients show more cortisol suppression than normal controls

C. The test has a specificity around 25% to 40% for diagnosing depression

D. Patients with a positive test may respond better to ECT than those with a negative test

E. Dexamethasone suppression is not routinely used as a clinical test for depression

61. **Which of the following is an advantage of using CT scan over MRI scan for diagnostic purposes?**
    A. Finer details are seen easily with CT scan
    B. Absence of radiation exposure in CT scan
    C. CT scan is more suitable in pregnant women
    D. CT scan is more immediately available in emergencies
    E. Anterior fossa is better visualized with CT scan

62. **Choose one of the following conditions where CT scan of brain is the investigation of choice**
    A. Subarachnoid haemorrhage
    B. Demyelinating disease
    C. Meningeal neoplasm
    D. Viral meningitis
    E. Ischaemic infarction of cortex

63. **A patient with bipolar disorder recently stabilized on medications is brought to you with a history of fever for 4 days and blurred vision, muscle fasciculation, hyperactive tendon reflexes, and persistent nausea and vomiting for the last 2 days. Which one of the following may be implicated?**
    A. Haloperidol
    B. Lithium
    C. Valproate
    D. Clonazepam
    E. Carbamazepine

64. **A patient who has chronic schizophrenia is on a depot antipsychotic medication. Your consultant asks for an ECG. Which of the following will be of most interest to him?**
    A. PR interval
    B. RR interval
    C. U waves
    D. QT interval
    E. Axis of heart

65. **Which of the following medications has the highest propensity to cause QT prolongation on ECG?**
    A. Thioridazine
    B. Risperidone
    C. Quetiapine
    D. Haloperidol
    E. Olanzapine

66. **A patient who is on olanzapine for a long time is developing xanthoma. Which one of the following levels might be elevated in his blood?**

A. Creatinine
B. Carotene
C. Cholesterol
D. Glucose
E. Albumin

67. **Which of the following nutrients, if deficient, can make treatment of depression difficult?**

A. B_{12}
B. Riboflavin
C. Nicotinamide
D. Folate
E. Magnesium

68. **Which of the following is a good predictor of metabolic side-effects of antipsychotics?**

A. QT interval
B. Lipid levels
C. HbA1c
D. Waist circumference
E. Ear lobe thickness

69. **In patients with suspected dementia, which of the following neuroimaging modalities is clinically helpful to differentiate dementia of Lewy body type from Alzheimer's dementia?**

A. CT scan
B. Structural MRI scan
C. Functional MRI scan
D. Dopamine transporter SPECT scan
E. PET scan

70. **Which of the following EEG rhythms has the highest frequency?**

A. Beta
B. Theta
C. Alpha
D. Delta
E. Mu

71. **In patients with delirium due to hepatic failure which of the following EEG change may be seen?**
    A. Hypsarrythmia
    B. Spike and wave pattern
    C. Periodic complexes
    D. Sleep spindles
    E. Slow triphasic waves

72. **Which of the following suggests a successful seizure activity after ECT?**
    A. Ictal facilitation
    B. Postictal suppression
    C. Ictal suppression
    D. Dominant alpha waves
    E. See-saw pattern

73. **In neurological examination, which of the following is seen in hypothyroidism?**
    A. Hypertonia
    B. Loss of deep tendon reflexes
    C. Slow and sluggish deep tendon reflexes
    D. Clonus on testing deep tendon reflexes
    E. Exaggerated jaw jerk

74. **Which one of the following patients is not suitable for undergoing MRI investigation when required?**
    A. A 32-year-old woman with last menstrual period 3 months ago
    B. A 74-year-old man with suspected Lewy body dementia
    C. A 53-year-old man with a cardiac pacemaker inserted 10 years ago
    D. A 44-year-old lady with a family history of haemochromatosis
    E. A 22-year-old man with epilepsy and mild learning disability

75. **Which of the following is the most clinically useful method of diagnosing Alzheimer's disease?**
    A. Clinical interview
    B. CT scans
    C. Functional MRI
    D. SPECT
    E. Lumbar puncture

1. A.   Questions used in clinical interviews can be either facilitative or obstructive. Facilitative messages help the interview to flow, establish a rapport and gain the confidence of the patient. For example, open-ended questions, facilitating statements, reflections, silence, interpretations, positive reinforcements, etc. Run on or polythematic questioning refers to the process of asking the patient a number of questions at the same time. For example, 'Have you felt high in spirits, gone on spending sprees and made foolish investments in the past week?' These questions can be obstructive. Self disclosures are statements about oneself (the psychiatrist) that may help establish a rapport with the patient. I want messages are generally used when the interview fails to progress because the patient is stuck on the same topic. In this case, the psychiatrist could say politely that he or she wants to move on to other topics.

Hales R and Yudofsky SC, eds. *The American Psychiatric Publishing Textbook of Clinical Psychiatry*. American Psychiatric Press, 2003, pp.166–171.

2. B.   Open-ended questions reflect a topic that the psychiatrist may want to explore, but leaves it open to the patient to say what he/she thinks is important. These questions are used to start the interview and, later on, can lead to specific closed-ended questions. Put down questions are where the underlying message is a criticism. For example 'How can you complain when you have got an A grade in your GCSE?' Facilitation statements encourage the patient to continue along a particular line of thought. For example, statements such as 'Go on'; 'Proceed'; 'What else' are facilitation statements.

Hales R and Yudofsky SC, eds. *The American Psychiatric Publishing Textbook of Clinical Psychiatry*. American Psychiatric Press, 2003, pp.166–171.

3. A.   A question whose answer cannot be a simple yes or no, or a single factual answer that can be classified as right or wrong, is an open-ended question, such as the question given in 3. A. (See also Question 2).

Kay J and Tasman A. *Essentials of Psychiatry*. John Wiley & Sons, 2006, p. 44.

4. E.   Reflections are statements where the psychiatrist repeats what the patient has just said. This gives an opportunity to correct one's understanding of what the patient said and to let the patient know that the clinician is listening and trying to understand the situation the patient is in. Interpretations are inferences reached by examining patterns of behaviour or thoughts expressed at a clinical interview.

Hales R and Yudofsky SC, eds. *The American Psychiatric Publishing Textbook of Clinical Psychiatry*. American Psychiatric Press, 2003, pp.166–171.

5. B.   Directiveness in the interview ensures that a clinician has all the information needed from a patient. Highly directive intervention aims to focus and restrict the patient's speech content and behaviour. These may include check lists or yes/no questions. Limit setting and redirection include situations where a clinician attempts to change the direction of the interview, especially when the interview is not progressing in the detail of information transferred.

Kay J and Tasman A. *Essentials of Psychiatry*. John Wiley & Sons, 2006, p. 44.

6. B.   Being empathetic and acknowledging a patient's emotional state helps in facilitating progression of clinical interview. These are supportive interventions required in various degrees by patients. Summarization is not an intervention but a technique facilitating a clinician's understanding of a patient's story. Confrontation may be helpful in some situations, but it cannot be considered as a supportive intervention during clinical interview.

Kay J and Tasman A. *Essentials of Psychiatry*. John Wiley & Sons, 2006, p. 44.

7. D.   Thoughts of self harm should always be enquired about. Contemplation of suicide is very common among the mentally ill. There is no evidence that enquiring about suicidal ideations increases the risk of committing suicide. In fact many patients would welcome an opportunity to discuss any suicidal thoughts with a professional.

Semple DM *et al.*, eds. *Oxford Handbook of Psychiatry*, 1st edn. Oxford University Press, 2005, p. 45.

8. B.   First rank symptoms (FRS), proposed by Kurt Schneider, suggest a diagnosis of schizophrenia. These symptoms are not specific for schizophrenia. The prevalence of FRS in schizophrenia ranges from 28% to 72%. First rank symptoms do not carry any prognostic significance. The stated question in this case enquires for the presence of 'running commentary' hallucinations – voices commenting on patients' thoughts or actions. Bleuler's primary or fundamental symptoms consist of loosening of association, blunting of affect, ambivalence, and autism (the four A's). All delusions and hallucinations were classed as secondary symptoms according to Bleuler. Negative symptoms include alogia, affective flattening, avolition, apathy, anhedonia, asociality, and attentional impairment.

Semple DM *et al.*, eds. *Oxford Handbook of Psychiatry*, 1st edn. Oxford University Press, 2005, p. 179.

9. A.   While administering the MMSE, the subject is asked to guess the answer if he is unsure. This could possibly differentiate patients with pseudodementia who usually answer 'I don't know' while truly demented patients often give wrong responses. On the attention subtest, initially the patient is asked to do the serial seven. If the score is less than 5, we do the WORLD backwards. The higher score among the two is taken. It is not enough for the patient to read the sentence out loud. It is a test of comprehension, so the patient needs to close his/her eyes after reading the command. Education affects the scores on the MMSE. Patients with higher educational status tend to score higher on the test. But education does not affect the rate of change of scores in both normal and dementia subject, and hence change in scores is a good index of worsening dementia. MMSE is not independent of socioeconomic status. This may be because socioeconomic status is indirectly linked to educational status.

Ridha B and Rossor M. The Mini Mental State Examination. *Practical Neurology* 2005; **5**: 298–303.

10. E.   The three dimensions of insight proposed by David include: the ability to label unusual experiences as pathological, to recognize that one has mental illness, and to comply with treatment. In a different approach to the concept of insight, emotional insight is considered the highest level of insight. This is the awareness and understanding of the illness which leads to a change in behaviour. Intellectual insight is the admission of illness and recognition of symptoms, without the ability to apply this knowledge to change or shape future behaviour. Patients with OCD may present with poor insight. DSM IV has a specifier 'with poor insight' for OCD where poor insight is associated with poor prognosis. Patients with schizophrenia show variable levels of insight at various stages of their illness. Some exhibit a good level of insight when recovered, while at the worst phase of their illness they may deny having any mental illness.

Sadock BJ and Sadock VA. *Kaplan & Sadock's Synopsis of Psychiatry: Behavioral Sciences/Clinical Psychiatry*, 10th edn. Lippincott Williams & Wilkins, 2007, p. 241.

11. E.   Option A and B indicate collusion with the patient's belief. Option C is a direct confrontation while D is evasion from the topic which can reduce engagement.

Semple DM *et al.*, eds. *Oxford Handbook of Psychiatry*, 1st edn. Oxford University Press, 2005, p. 56.

12. A.   Childhood physical, sexual abuse, and neglect are extremely common experiences among those who develop serious mental health problems. But victims are typically reluctant to disclose their histories of abuse and psychiatrists are often reluctant to seek this important information. Though clinicians are not comfortable exploring sexual abuse in the first interview, postponing the discussion once it is disclosed is not an advisable strategy.

Read J, *et al.* Why, when and how to ask about childhood abuse. *Advances in Psychiatric Treatment* 2007; **13**: 101–110.

13. C.   While interviewing people with limited intelligence, questions should be brief and worded in a simple way. Closed and leading questions are best avoided as suggestibility is prominent in this population. Suggestibility in patients with limited intelligence can be assessed using the Gudjonnson Suggestibility Scale. Closed questions are a good way of eliciting information from a disturbed psychotic patient who is guarded or distracted by hallucinations. Confrontation through closed questions may be useful in malingerers.

Gudjonsson GH and Henry L. Child and adult witnesses with intellectual disability: The importance of suggestibility. *Legal and Criminological Psychology* 2003; **8**: 241–252.

14. E.   There is no single question that can reliably elicit premorbid personality traits. A detailed discourse that includes enquiry about hobbies, leisure, predominant mood state, character, and descriptions – both self and by friends – is necessary to understand one's premorbid personality.

Sadock BJ and Sadock VA. *Kaplan & Sadock's Synopsis of Psychiatry: Behavioral Sciences/Clinical Psychiatry*, 10th edn. Lippincott Williams & Wilkins, 2007, p. 228.

15. D.   The CAGE questionnaire includes questions on 'Cut down', 'Annoyed', 'Guilty', and 'Eye opener'. Early morning drinking (not evening as indicated in the question) indicates a problem use of alcohol.

Semple DM *et al.*, eds. *Oxford Handbook of Psychiatry*, 1st edn. Oxford University Press, 2005, p. 509.

16. E.   While self neglect can be seen in any severe mental illness, it is not very common in isolated anxiety disorders. In alcoholism self neglect indicates a higher risk of vitamin and nutritional deficiencies. In schizophrenia, this may be secondary to negative symptoms or depression.

Garden G. Physical examination in psychiatric practice. *Advances in Psychiatric Treatment* 2005; **11**: 142–149.

17. A. Exuberant dressing and makeup suggests elevated mood. It is possible that the lady described in this scenario has bipolar illness.

Semple DM *et al.*, eds. *Oxford Handbook of Psychiatry*, 1st edn. Oxford University Press, 2005, p. 38.

18. B. Serial sevens test is a part of Mini Mental State Examination. In this test, the subject is asked to subtract seven from 100 serially for five times. One point is given for each correct subtraction. Though it has arithmetic properties, in MMSE this test is primarily administered to test attention. Alternatively, the subject may be asked to spell the word 'WORLD' backwards to test attention. The better of two scores is used to calculate final MMSE scores.

Ridha B and Rossor M. The Mini Mental State Examination. *Practical Neurology* 2005; **5**: 298–303.

19. D. Hallucinatory behaviours, such as the one described in this example, are often noted in acutely psychotic patients with poor insight. Questioning the behaviour gently could elicit more information from the patient.

Semple DM *et al.*, eds. *Oxford Handbook of Psychiatry*, 1st edn. Oxford University Press, 2005, p. 38.

20. B. Reactivity of affect refers to change in affect in response to environmental cues. Lack of reactivity is common in depression. Congruity is the appropriateness of the person's affect to the symptoms or the thought content. In this case, the affect is appropriate to the symptom of depression.

Semple DM *et al.*, eds. *Oxford Handbook of Psychiatry*, 1st edn. Oxford University Press, 2005, p. 81.

21. A. Stability of affect refers to maintaining a particular affective state for a reasonable period of time. Unstable or labile affect – when extreme – presents as emotional incontinence seen in stroke. Severe lability of affect seen in stroke, especially in pseudobulbar palsy, is also called the PLAC (pathological laughter and crying) syndrome. Labile affect is also a feature of mania and delirium.

Sadock BJ and Sadock VA. *Kaplan & Sadock's Synopsis of Psychiatry: Behavioral Sciences/Clinical Psychiatry*, 10th edn. Lippincott Williams & Wilkins, 2007, p. 233.

22. E. Various schools of thought exist in distinguishing mood from affect. It is generally accepted that mood refers to a more pervasive emotional state than affect. (Climate = mood vs. weather = affect!) Both mood and affect can have objective and subjective components though one school maintains that mood is subjective while affect is objective.

Semple DM *et al.*, eds. *Oxford Handbook of Psychiatry*, 1st edn. Oxford University Press, 2005, pp. 82, 96.
Sadock BJ and Sadock VA. *Kaplan & Sadock's Synopsis of Psychiatry: Behavioral Sciences/Clinical Psychiatry*, 10th edn. Lippincott Williams & Wilkins, 2007, p. 241.

23. A. Nihilism is similar to pessimism with self reference of an extreme belief, for example 'My brain is rotten'. Congruence refers to 'in keeping with' a particular state of mind – nihilism is usually congruent with depression. Nihilism with delusional intensity is seen in psychotic depression.

Semple DM *et al.*, eds. *Oxford Handbook of Psychiatry*, 1st edn. Oxford University Press, 2005, p. 96.

24. E. Direct questioning about suicidality does not increase risk of suicide, so evasive questioning is not recommended. A step-wise approach, starting from enquiry about mood state, hopelessness and thoughts of death, passive wishes to die, and active suicidal plans, is often useful in assessment of suicidal thoughts.

Semple DM *et al.*, eds. *Oxford Handbook of Psychiatry*, 1st edn. Oxford University Press, 2005, p. 45

25. B.   Features suggestive of hypothyroidism include, slowing of EEG, excessive daytime sleepiness, hypothermia, cerebellar ataxia, dementia, psychosis. The peripheral neuropathy in hypothyroidism is a sensorimotor polyneuropathy with loss of reflexes, diminution in vibratory, joint position, and touch–pressure sensations, and weakness in the distal parts of the limbs. Myopathy may also be present. Nerve conduction studies typically show a slowing of nerve conduction velocities. Hypothyroidism is observed to be common in patients with Down's syndrome.

Ropper AH and Brown RH, eds. *Adams and Victor's Principles of Neurology,* 8th edn. McGraw-Hill Companies, 2005, p. 1151.

26. C.   Russell's sign was first described in bulimia nervosa. This refers to the skin abrasions, on the dorsum of the hand overlying the fingers, found in patients with symptoms of bulimia. These are caused by repeated contact between the incisors and the skin of the hand which occurs during self-induced vomiting.

Semple DM *et al.,* eds. *Oxford Handbook of Psychiatry,* 1st edn. Oxford University Press, 2005, p. 99.

27. B.   These features are suggestive of opiate withdrawal. Classical withdrawal from opiates appears in 4 to 12 hours, peaks in 48 to 72 hours, and subsides in a week. It is characterized by symptoms of muscle aches and cramps, severe anxiety and agitation, insomnia, diarrhoea, shivering, yawning, and fatigue. Signs include tachycardia and hypertension, lacrimation, rhinorrhoea, dilated pupils, and 'goose-fleshing' (piloerection) of the skin (hence 'cold turkey' or 'clucking'). Insomnia (with increase in REM sleep) and craving for the drug may persist for weeks. Opiate withdrawal is not usually life threatening.

Gelder MG *et al.,* eds. *New Oxford Textbook of Psychiatry.* Oxford University Press, 2000, p. 524.

28. C.   The features of acute confusion, nystagmus, ocular palsy, and ataxia are suggestive of Wernicke's encephalopathy, possibly secondary to alcohol use in a 50-year-old male. In females, an additional likely cause of Wernicke's encephalopathy is hyperemesis secondary to pregnancy or anorexia. Wernicke's encephalopathy is an indirect result of thiamine deficiency. It may be precipitated on administration of glucose to a confused patient in the casualty department. Glucose causes a sudden depletion of the available thiamine stores (via thiamine-dependent transketolase). In people recovering from Wernicke's encephalopathy, 80% develop a Korsakoff's syndrome which is characterized by deficits in anterograde and retrograde memory, apathy, an intact sensorium, and relative preservation of other intellectual abilities.

Gelder MG *et al.,* eds. *New Oxford Textbook of Psychiatry.* Oxford University Press, 2000, p. 460.

29. C.   The clinical situation given here is an example of an acute dystonic reaction in a young male, possibly a psychotic patient, who has been started on an antipsychotic. Given the options, risperidone is the most likely causative agent. Procyclidine may relieve the dystonic attack. Alternatively, a benzodiazepine or an antihistamine with anticholinergic action may be used. Risk factors of dystonia include male gender, age younger than 30 years, and using high dosages of high-potency, typical antipsychotics.

Semple DM *et al.,* eds. *Oxford Handbook of Psychiatry,* 1st edn. Oxford University Press, 2005, p. 866.

30. A.   Absence of nystagmus during an attack of dizziness almost always rules out vertigo secondary to labyrinthine or brain stem pathology. The dizziness here is most likely to be psychogenic in origin – related to panic attacks. This may be accompanied by agoraphobia, which is described as a fear of being in places from where escape may seem impossible or difficult.

Kasper DL, *et al.,* eds. *Harrison's Principles of Internal Medicine,* 16th edn. McGraw-Hill Companies, 2005, p. 132.

31. E.   The onset of Huntington's disease is invariably insidious and gradually progressing. Acute onset of chorea is suggestive of a metabolic cause or secondary to toxins. Huntington's disease is an autosomal dominant disease with full penetrance, that is every person with the mutant gene will develop the full form of the disease if they live long enough. Huntington's disease also exhibits genetic anticipation, that is each successive generation suffers progressively earlier onset. Huntington's is a disease of trinucleotide repeat sequences in genetic coding. The pathogenesis is an excess CAG repeats in the *IT15* gene on chromosome 4p. The age of onset depends on the actual number of trinucleotide repeats. Symptoms of Huntington's disease consist of a triad – motor, cognitive, and psychiatric problems. The prevalence of Huntington's is around 4–7 per 100,000 with average life expectancy less than 15 years after symptomatic clinical presentation.

Kasper DL, et al., eds. *Harrison's Principles of Internal Medicine*, 16th edn. McGraw-Hill Companies, 2005, p. 139.

32. A.   Features suggestive of subacute combined degeneration of the cord (SACD) include paraesthesias, difficulties with gait and balance, and signs of posterior column dysfunction. This results in sensory ataxia with a positive Romberg's sign and bladder atony. Pain and temperature sensations are usually intact. Bilateral corticospinal tract dysfunction in SACD results in spasticity, hyper-reflexia, and bilateral Babinski's signs. However, reflexes may be lost or hypoactive because of superimposed peripheral neuropathy.

Brazis P, et al. *Localisation in Clinical Neurology*, 5th edn. Lippincott Williams & Wilkins, 2007, p. 106.

33. E.   Factitious disorder is a condition where clinical symptoms are consciously and intentionally produced by the patient. But interestingly the only gain for the patient from such symptom production is the adoption of a patient's role, without any clear monetary or employment gains. In malingering, symptoms are consciously and intentionally produced, but the goal is a material or concrete gain, for example claiming employment compensation or avoiding military duty. In somatoform disorders, such as somatization, the symptoms are not produced intentionally and the origin remains unconscious.

Sadock BJ and Sadock VA. *Kaplan & Sadock's Synopsis of Psychiatry: Behavioral Sciences/Clinical Psychiatry*, 10th edn. Lippincott Williams & Wilkins, 2007, p. 660.

34. B.   Neuroleptic malignant syndrome is a medical emergency that can occur when treating a patient with antipsychotics. Symptoms and signs include muscular rigidity, altered consciousness, akinesia, mutism, and agitation. Autonomic symptoms include hyperthermia (temperature >38°C), sweating, labile pulse rate, and fluctuating blood pressure. Altered consciousness is not seen in tardive dyskinesia or akathisia.

Semple DM et al., eds. *Oxford Handbook of Psychiatry*, 1st edn. Oxford University Press, 2005, p. 868.

35. C.   General health questionnaire (GHQ) is used to define psychiatric 'caseness' in epidemiological studies. In community surveys where a large population is screened, the best technique to detect psychiatric illness consists of two phases. Initially, potential cases are identified using a self-rated questionnaire, such as GHQ. Once 'caseness' is suspected, detailed interviews or other diagnostic tools are used to confirm a diagnosis. MMPI stands for Minnesota Multiphasic Personality Inventory. It is a detailed questionnaire used to measure various personality traits (not disorders). HDRS stands for Hamilton Depression Rating Scale. It is a commonly used, clinician administered mood rating scale after a diagnosis of depression is made. Young's Mania Rating Scale (YMRS) is used to measure severity of mania or hypomania.

Goldberg DP, et al. *Manual of the General Health Questionnaire*. NFER Publishing, Windsor, England, 1978.

36. E. Argyll Robertson pupil (ARP) is characteristically associated with neurosyphilis. It refers to bilaterally irregular and miotic pupils with variable iris atrophy. It is also characterized by light near dissociation in which light reflex is absent but accommodation reflex is intact. The site of the lesion causing ARP is the rostral midbrain. There are a number of conditions, including long-standing diabetes, that can cause light near dissociation. Normally, pupils dilate in darkness. In Flynn phenomenon, paradoxically, pupils constrict in darkness. This is seen in congenital achromatopsia, dominant optic atrophy, and in some cases with congenital nystagmus.

Brazis P, et al. Localisation in Clinical Neurology, 5th edn. Lippincott Williams & Wilkins, 2007, p. 203.

37. A. Thunderclap headaches are sudden onset, severe headaches radiating behind the occiput with some degree of associated neck stiffness. Very rarely a thunderclap variant of migraine may be seen. This needs to be differentiated from an intracranial bleed. Tension headache is suggested by generalized or bilateral, continuous, tight band-like pain which worsens as the day progresses. It is associated with stress and is often aggravated by eye movement. It is usually relieved by simple analgesics or antidepressants. Migraine is suggested by a typically unilateral, throbbing headache associated with vomiting, prodromal aura, and visual disturbances. Migraine is often precipitated by a set of well-known precipitating factors such as chocolates, menstruation, etc, which most patients will learn during the course of their illness. A cluster headache is suggested by episodic, typically nocturnal pain in one eye associated with congestion and lacrimation for weeks. This cyclically recurs every year at around the same time. Temporal arteritis is suggested by scalp tenderness, jaw claudication, loss of temporal arterial pulsation, sudden loss of vision, and a raised ESR. It is confirmed by temporal artery biopsy.

Douglas G, et al., eds. Macleod's Clinical Examination, 11th edn. Churchill Livingstone, 2005, p. 229.

38. A. Waddling gait is seen with severe proximal muscle weakness. Weakness of gluteus medius results in an excessive drop of the hip bone towards the side opposite to the foot placement. Corticospinal tract lesions give rise to a spastic gait. This can be hemiparetic when the lesion is unilateral and paraparetic when the lesion is bilateral. Cerebellar lesions cause a complex gait disturbance according to the area affected. Unsteadiness on standing with eyes open is suggestive of cerebellar lesion. Cerebellar dysfunction leads to a broad-based, unsteady (drunken or ataxic) gait. Postural instability that becomes prominent on closure of eyes is indicative of proprioceptive sensory loss, referred to as sensory ataxia. In order to maintain a stable posture, at least two out of three sources of sensory information regarding one's posture should be normal, that is visual input, vestibular input, and joint position sense. When joint position sense is lost due to posterior column lesion, closing one's eyes will prevent the visual input from compensating for the deficit, leading to loss of balance. 'Astasia abasia' is a conversion disorder where the gait does not confirm to any known neurological deficits. Sometimes such a patient can walk normally but cannot stand and balance herself without support.

Brazis P, et al. Localisation in Clinical Neurology, 5th edn. Lippincott Williams & Wilkins, 2007, p. 238.

39. B. Bilateral upper motor neurone lesions of the corticobulbar tract result in pseudobulbar or spastic dysarthria. This is characterized by a small, spastic tongue and difficulty pronouncing consonants. It is associated with pathological laughing and crying. Bulbar palsy is the result of lower motor neurone lesions affecting the nuclei of cranial nerves. The extent of speech disturbance in bulbar palsy depends on the specific cranial nerves involved. Extrapyramidal dysarthria is characterized by a loss in prosody as seen in Parkinson's disease, while cerebellar dysarthria refers to slurred drunken-like speech in patients with cerebellar ataxia. Myasthenia gravis is associated with speech that deteriorates in tone and strength during a discourse secondary to muscular fatigue.

Douglas G, et al., eds. Macleod's Clinical Examination, 11th edn. Churchill Livingstone, 2005, p. 239.

40. B.   Apraxia is defined as the inability to carry out a motor act despite the absence of sensory or motor deficits. Here the muscular power and tone will be intact and the patient can fully comprehend the instruction. There are many classifications of apraxia according to region affected, for example oculomotor, orofacial, limb-kinetic apraxia. Apraxia is also classified according to specific functional defect, for example dressing apraxia, constructional apraxia, etc. With the exception of dressing and constructional apraxia, apraxic abnormalities are usually secondary to left hemisphere damage. In particular, this includes injuries involving the left frontal and inferior parietal lobes. Ideomotor apraxia (IMA) is the most common type of apraxia. Patients with ideomotor apraxia usually struggle with imitation and copying of skilled movements and falter when using tools. When pantomiming the use of a screwdriver, patients with ideomotor apraxia may rotate their arm at the shoulder and fix their elbow.

Bradley GW, *et al.*, eds. *Neurology in Clinical Practice*, 4th edn. Butterworth-Heineman, 2003, pp. 117–131.

41. A.   Ideational apraxia is an inability to correctly sequence a series of goal-directed acts in spite of the ability to execute the instructions when broken down into single acts. Asking the patient to demonstrate how to prepare a sandwich for lunch is a good test of ideational apraxia because it tests for a sequence of acts. Ideational apraxia is most often associated with dementia. Patients with conceptual apraxia suffer from difficulty in understanding the concept of using tools. Hence they will fail in tests for ideomotor apraxia. Unlike patients with conceptual apraxia, those with ideomotor apraxia have preserved concepts of using tools, but they cannot perform the action when required. Patients with limb-kinetic apraxia demonstrate a loss of dexterity and ability to make finely graded, precise, independent finger movements. They will not be able to employ pincer grasp to pick up a penny. They will also have trouble rotating a coin between the thumb, middle finger, and little finger. Limb-kinetic apraxia most often occurs in the limb contralateral to a hemispheric lesion.

Bradley GW, *et al.*, eds. *Neurology in Clinical Practice*, 4th edn. Butterworth-Heineman, 2003, pp. 117–131.

42. A.   Pure word deafness is a syndrome of isolated loss of auditory comprehension and repetition, without any abnormality of speech, naming, reading, or writing. Pure word deafness is caused by bilateral or sometimes unilateral lesion, isolating Wernicke's area from the input of both Heschl's gyri. Wernicke's aphasia presents with logorrhoea, neologisms, and paragrammatism. Most patients have no elementary motor or sensory deficits. It may be associated with right homonymous hemianopia or upper quandrantanopia. The language disturbances seen in Wernicke's aphasia may be difficult to distinguish from those of schizophrenia. People with Broca's aphasia show agrammatism. Reading is often impaired in Broca's aphasia despite preserved auditory comprehension. It is associated with right hemiparesis, hemisensory loss, and apraxia of the non-paralysed left limbs. Patients with motor aphasia have higher risk of depression. In transcortical aphasia the features of Broca's and Wernicke's aphasias are combined but with intact repetition. Lesions producing transcortical aphasia disrupt connections from other cortical centres into the language circuit. Anomic aphasia refers to an aphasic syndrome wherein naming is the principal deficit. Anomic aphasia is related to dominant angular gyrus lesion and may be accompanied by dominant parietal lesions.

Bradley GW, *et al.*, eds. *Neurology in Clinical Practice*, 4th edn. Butterworth-Heineman, 2003, pp. 141–161.

43. A. Alexia is the acquired inability to read. Alexia with agraphia is seen in angular gyrus lesions and is associated with Gerstmann syndrome. Alexia with agraphia is seen in insufficiency of vascular supply to territories of angular branch of middle cerebral artery. Patients with alexia without agraphia can write reasonably but cannot read written language. Left posterior cerebral artery insufficiency is associated with alexia without agraphia. This leads to infarction of the medial occipital lobe, the splenium of the corpus callosum, and often extending to the medial temporal lobe. Comprehension is preserved in conduction aphasia. In global aphasia, speech production will be impaired. Conduction aphasia is a result of a lesion in the arcuate fasciculus. Writing and spontaneous reading (not repetition) is preserved in isolated conduction aphasia.

Bradley GW, *et al.*, eds. *Neurology in Clinical Practice*, 4th edn. Butterworth-Heineman, 2003, pp. 141–161.

44. E. Muscle atrophy, fasciculations, absent reflexes, and hypotonia are features suggestive of lower motor neurone lesion. Features suggestive of upper motor neurone lesion include absence of fasciculations, hypertonia, minimal wasting of muscles, and exaggerated deep tendon reflexes. Corticobulbar and corticospinal tracts are the major upper motor neurone tracts while all peripheral and cranial nerves with motor components perform lower motor neurone function.

Douglas G, *et al.*, eds. *Macleod's Clinical Examination*, 11th edn. Churchill Livingstone, 2005, p. 269.

45. A. Cerebellar limb ataxia is characterized by dysmetria (past pointing), intention tremor, dysdiadochokinesia, and excessive rebound of outstretched arms against a resistance that is suddenly removed. It is also associated with hypotonia and pendular deep tendon reflexes. Asymmetric cerebellar pathology can cause lateralized imbalance with nystagmus, which is present even when eyes are open. This is not Romberg's sign. Romberg's sign refers to prominent postural instability in patients with dorsal spinal column damage when attempting to stand with eyes shut.

Kasper DL, *et al.*, eds. *Harrison's Principles of Internal Medicine*, 16th edn. McGraw-Hill Companies, 2005, p. 140.

46. B. Brown–Sequard syndrome is the result of hemisection of the spinal cord. This consists of: (1) loss of contralateral pain and temperature due to interruption of the crossed spinothalamic tract and (2) loss of ipsilateral proprioception below the level of the lesion due to involvement of the ascending fibres in the posterior columns. It is also associated with ipsilateral spastic weakness due to involvement of the descending corticospinal tract. The 'sensory level' is usually one or two segments below the level of the lesion.

Brazis P, *et al. Localisation in Clinical Neurology*, 5th edn. Lippincott Williams & Wilkins, 2007, p. 105.

47. B. Lid retraction is the most common clinical feature of Grave's ophthalmopathy. The associated extraocular myopathy is attributed to inflammation and fibrosis of muscles. Inferior rectus is most commonly involved and lateral rectus is the least involved of all extraocular muscles. Diplopia may be especially worse early in the day. Other signs include orbital congestion, lid lag on looking down, proptosis, conjunctival injection, and optic neuropathy due to compression of the optic nerve by enlarged extraocular muscles in the orbital apex.

Brazis P, *et al. Localisation in Clinical Neurology*, 5th edn. Lippincott Williams & Wilkins, 2007, p. 175.

48. C. Cluster headache is considered as a vascular headache syndrome. It is usually episodic in nature and is characterized by attacks of acute, periorbital pain. This pain is often deep and excruciating but rarely pulsatile. It occurs almost every day over a 4–8 week period, followed by a pain-free interval that averages a year. Attacks last from 30 minutes to 2 hours. It is often associated with lacrimation, reddening of the eye, nasal stuffiness, lid ptosis, and nausea. It is common in men aged 20 to 50 years. Propranolol and amitriptyline are ineffective. Lithium is beneficial for cluster headache though ineffective for migraine.

Kasper DL, *et al.*, eds. *Harrison's Principles of Internal Medicine*, 16th edn. McGraw-Hill, 2005, p. 93.

49. B. Tuberous sclerosis is a congenital disease where hyperplasia of ectodermal and mesodermal cells leads to various lesions in the skin, nervous system, heart, kidney and other organs. It is characterized clinically by the triad of adenoma sebaceum, epilepsy, and mental retardation. Hypomelanotic skin macules (ash-leaf lesions) and subepidermal fibroses (shagreen patches) are other associated skin lesions noted in tuberous sclerosis. Neurofibromatosis is a hereditary neoplastic syndrome where benign tumours of the skin, nervous system, bones, and endocrine organs are seen. Café au lait spots are characteristic, coffee-coloured skin patches seen in neurofibromatosis. In Sturge–Weber syndrome (encephalotrigeminal angiomatosis), facial port wine stain associated with cerebral angiomatosis is seen. Fabry's disease is a glycogen storage disease.

Ropper AH and Brown RH, eds. *Adams and Victor's Principles of Neurology*, 8th edn. McGraw-Hill Companies, 2005, p. 865.

50. D. Progressive supranuclear palsy is a degenerative neurological disease with parkinsonian symptoms as a prominent clinical feature. It is characterized by axial akinetic rigidity, dizziness, unsteadiness, falls, and pseudobulbar dysarthria. Eye movement abnormalities affecting down gaze occur first, followed by variable limitations of upward and horizontal eye movement. Doll's eye movements are preserved as the brain stem is intact. Upper motor neurone signs and occasionally cerebellar signs may be present. Dementia is a common sequel.

Kasper DL, *et al.*, eds. *Harrison's Principles of Internal Medicine*, 16th edn. McGraw-Hill, 2005, p. 2414.

51. B. Trigeminal neuralgia is characterized by episodic shooting pain in facial areas supplied by trigeminal nerve. It often follows specific sensory triggers in the trigeminal zone, for example shaving one's beard, brushing teeth, etc. It is often idiopathic though at times cases of arteriovenous malformations in brainstem around the site where the trigeminal nerve exits the brain stem have been found. An essential feature of trigeminal neuralgia is that objective signs of sensory loss cannot be demonstrated on examination. All the other choices present with trigeminal neuropathy, which is characterized by an objective sign of sensory loss in the distribution of the division of the trigeminal nerve involved.

Kasper DL, *et al.*, eds. *Harrison's Principles of Internal Medicine*, 16th edn. McGraw-Hill, 2005, p. 2434.

52. E. Causes of bilateral facial palsy include granulomatous and connective tissue diseases such as systemic lupus erythematosus, Sjögren's syndrome, sarcoidosis; infections such as meningitis, encephalitis, mastoiditis, leprosy; neoplasms, including pontine glioma and meningioma; trauma resulting in fracture of the temporal bone and birth injury. Miscellaneous known causes include prenatal exposure to thalidomide and chronic diabetes.

Brazis P, *et al*. *Localisation in Clinical Neurology*, 5th edn. Lippincott Williams & Wilkins, 2007, p. 296.

53. C. Lithium toxicity results in two major groups of symptoms – neurological and gastrointestinal. Delayed ankle jerk is secondary to hypothyroidism. Hypothyroidism in lithium users correlates with pre-existent tendency to develop antithyroid antibodies. This is not dependent on the dose of lithium administered. Coarse (4 to 7 Hz) rather than fine (8 to 12 Hz) tremors indicate lithium toxicity. The fine postural tremor associated with lithium therapy decreases with longer duration of treatment. Alopecia is independent of serum lithium levels.

Sadock BJ and Sadock VA. *Kaplan & Sadock's Synopsis of Psychiatry: Behavioral Sciences/Clinical Psychiatry*, 10th edn. Lippincott Williams & Wilkins, 2007, p. 1060.

54. A. Lanugo hair is thin, infantile hair noted on the torso and limbs of severely anorexic patient. Alopecia areata is an autoimmune skin lesion.

Sadock BJ and Sadock VA. *Kaplan & Sadock's Synopsis of Psychiatry: Behavioral Sciences/Clinical Psychiatry*, 10th edn. Lippincott Williams & Wilkins, 2007, p. 731.

55. C. During sleep, the body goes through two types of physiological states. This has been divided into REM and NREM phase according to EEG studies. NREM is further divided into four stages. At stage 1 smaller slower waves of theta frequency are noted. Stage 2 consists of K complexes and sleep spindles. Stages 3 and 4 are called slow wave sleep as they show dominant delta activity. Stage 3 consists of less than 50% delta activity while stage 4 consists of more than 50% delta waves. REM sleep is comprised of saw-tooth activity. In adults, 75% of sleep is NREM.

Sadock BJ and Sadock VA. *Kaplan & Sadock's Synopsis of Psychiatry: Behavioral Sciences/Clinical Psychiatry*, 10th edn. Lippincott Williams & Wilkins, 2007, p. 751.

56. E. An electroencephalograph represents cerebral cortical activity. EEG depends on afferent neural inputs from subcortical structures, including the thalamus and brainstem reticular formation. The thalamic afferents to the cortex are responsible for the alpha rhythm and sleep spindles usually seen in the second stage of NREM sleep. EEG is rarely specific to an illness because different conditions often produce non-specific and similar changes. Hypsarrythmia is associated with infantile spasms (West's syndrome). Three-Hz spike-and-wave activity is associated with typical absence attacks. Generalized multiple spikes and waves (poly-spike wave) are associated with myoclonic epilepsy. Certain parts of the cerebral cortex, such as inferior temporal lobe, are inaccessible to routine electrode placement.

Bradley GW, *et al.*, eds. *Neurology in Clinical Practice*, 4th edn. Butterworth-Heineman, 2003, pp. 465–491.

57. D. This scenario depicts acute intermittent porphyria (AIP). It is one of the groups of disorders of haem metabolism, characterized by neurological and psychiatric manifestations without obvious cutaneous markers. AIP manifests itself by abdomen pain, neuropathies, and constipation, but, unlike most types of porphyria, patients with AIP do not have a rash. It is an autosomal dominant disorder with presentation starting between ages 18 and 40. It is episodic in nature and the episodes are often triggered by certain medications including oestrogens, barbiturates, and benzodiazepines. Diclofenac can precipitate an episode. Psychiatric manifestations include depression, anxiety, delirium, and psychosis. The most important lab. test is demonstrating increased urinary porphobilinogen during acute attacks. Treatment is aimed at reducing haem synthesis by administering haemin.

Anderson KE, *et al.* Recommendations for the diagnosis and treatment of the acute porphyrias. *Annals of Internal Medicine* 2005; **142**: 439–450.

58. E. All of these features except a history of seizure disorder may help to differentiate seizures from pseudoseizures. Pseudoseizures are more common in patients with epilepsy than those without. So having an established diagnosis of epilepsy does not rule out pseudoseizures. Patients with pseudoseizures do not have the characteristic prolactin elevation noted after an episode of true seizure; they may have unusually prolonged seizures with asymmetric limb involvement but without bladder or bowel control being lost.

Kasper DL, *et al.*, eds. *Harrison's Principles of Internal Medicine*, 16th edn. McGraw-Hill, 2005, p. 2366.

59. A. Incidence of agranulocytosis in patients on clozapine is less than 1 per 100 patients. The peak occurrence of agranulocytosis with clozapine is between 4 and 18 weeks after initiation of treatment. Weekly monitoring of the white cell or absolute neutrophil count is required for 18 to 26 weeks in most countries, with the frequency decreasing to biweekly or monthly thereafter. It is noted that the risk of clozapine-induced agranulocytosis is equivalent to the risk of agranulocytosis due to any other antipsychotic after 1 year of safe treatment. With regular monitoring, agranulocytosis can usually be detected before infection sets in. Discontinuation of clozapine, treatment with granulocyte colony stimulating factors, and vigorous treatment of infection are usually effective in restoring the white cell numbers. In UK, the Clozaril patient monitoring service (CPMS) maintains central laboratory data of all patients on Clozaril (generic form: clozapine) and sends one of three 'traffic light signals' to clinicians. Amber light is a sign of caution and a count should be repeated. With a red light, clozapine should be immediately stopped and re-challenge should not be done under normal circumstances.

Gelder MG *et al.*, eds. *New Oxford Textbook of Psychiatry*. Oxford University Press, 2000, 1319.

60. B. Exogenous administration of the steroid dexamethasone usually inhibits endogenous cortisol secretion. This cortisol suppression by the exogenous dexamethasone is impaired in patients with depression. This is thought to be due to a disturbed feedback mechanism among cortisol, adrenocorticotropic hormone (ACTH), and corticotrophin releasing hormone (CRH). Dexamethasone suppression is non-specific for depression and is also observed in patients with mania, schizophrenia, dementia, and other psychiatric disorders. There is some evidence to show that patients with dexamethasone non-suppression (test positive) respond well to physical interventions such as antidepressant therapy or electroconvulsive therapy compared to test negative population, though this is not widely replicated.

Sadock BJ and Sadock VA. *Kaplan & Sadock's Synopsis of Psychiatry: Behavioral Sciences/Clinical Psychiatry*, 10th edn. Lippincott Williams & Wilkins, 2007, 531.

61. D. Immediate availability, especially in head injury units, and ability to enable early detection of haemorrhages make CT scan the preferred diagnostic modality in emergency scenarios.

Kasper DL, *et al.*, eds. *Harrison's Principles of Internal Medicine*, 16th edn. McGraw-Hill Companies, 2005, 2350.

62. A. MRI is more sensitive than CT for the detection of lesions of the spinal cord, cranial nerves, and posterior fossa structures. Diffusion MR is the most sensitive technique for detecting acute ischemic stroke and is useful in the detection of encephalitis and abscesses. CT is the investigation of choice for suspected acute stroke, haemorrhage, and intracranial or spinal trauma. CT is also more sensitive than MRI for visualizing lesions of the bone.

Kasper DL, *et al.*, eds. *Harrison's Principles of Internal Medicine*, 16th edn. McGraw-Hill, 2005, p. 2350.

63. B. In this case, a patient's bipolar disorder has been stabilized on a particular medication. It is likely that this medication is lithium because the symptoms described here are consistent with lithium toxicity. This might have been precipitated by dehydration associated with fever. Other causes that may precipitate lithium toxicity are diarrhoeal illnesses, vomiting and fluid loss, and medications such as diuretics, NSAIDS and ACE inhibitors.

Sadock BJ and Sadock VA. *Kaplan & Sadock's Synopsis of Psychiatry: Behavioral Sciences/Clinical Psychiatry*, 10th edn. Lippincott Williams & Wilkins, 2007, p.1058.

64. D. Prolonged QT interval can predispose to serious ventricular arrhythmia called torsades de pointes (polymorphic ventricular arrhythmia). Many antipsychotics share the propensity to prolong QT interval. A troublesome change in heart rate is not observed clinically with most antipsychotics. Non-specific PR changes can occur with antipsychotic treatment.

Leonard BE. *Fundamentals of Psychopharmacology*, 3rd edn. Wiley, 2003, p. 293.

65. A. ECG abnormalities occur in approximately 25% of all patients on antipsychotics. The most commonly reported changes are the prolonged QT interval (suggestive of repolarization disturbances), depressed ST segments, and abnormal T waves. A prolonged QTc is more likely to be seen in patients with chronic schizophrenia treated with antipsychotics in doses greater than 200 mg chlorpromazine equivalents a day. Thioridazine, pimozide, sertindole, and droperidol prolong QT_C interval to a higher extent than other antipsychotics. TCAs share this propensity with antipsychotics. This predisposes to a fatal form of arrhythmia called torsades de pointes (polymorphic ventricular arrhythmia) leading to sudden death.

Leonard BE. *Fundamentals of Psychopharmacology*, 3rd edn. Wiley, 2003, p. 293.

66. C. Xanthomas indicate the presence of hyperlipidaemia. Metabolic syndrome is a common side-effect of atypical antipsychotic treatment. There is growing concern with metabolic disturbances associated with antipsychotic use, including hyperglycaemia, hyperlipidaemia, exacerbation of existing type 1 and 2 DM, new-onset type 2 DM, and diabetic ketoacidosis.

Chang HY *et al.* Eruptive xanthomas associated with olanzapine use. *Archives of Dermatology* 2003; **139**: 1045–1048.

67. D. Though folate deficiency itself is not a common cause of depression, in folate-deficient patients, supplementation might increase response to antidepressant treatment. It is currently not clear whether this effect is seen only in folate deficient individuals or if folate could be a potential adjuvant to antidepressant therapy in general.

Taylor MJ, Carney S, Geddes J, and Goodwin G. Folate for depressive disorders. *Cochrane Database Systematic Reviews* 2003; **2**: CD003390.

68. D. Waist circumference is a better predictor than baseline weight with respect to metabolic syndrome. HbA1c is not a screening measure. QT interval is unrelated to metabolic effects of antipsychotics. Here, metabolic side-effects refer to endocrine and metabolic changes associated with antipsychotic therapy.

Newcomer JW. Second-generation (atypical) antipsychotics and metabolic effects: a comprehensive literature review. *CNS Drugs* 2005; **19** (Suppl. 1): 1–93.

69. D. DAT (dopamine transporter) scan is a SPECT scan that visualizes dopamine transporter. Dementia with Lewy bodies (DLB) is one of the main differential diagnoses of Alzheimer's disease (AD). In DLB there is 40–70% loss of striatal dopamine and the loss of dopaminergic cell is accompanied by loss of the dopamine transporter. The loss of dopaminergic neurones in DLB can be confirmed *in vivo* with a DAT scan, which uses a radioligand that specifically binds to the dopamine transporter (FP-CIT). There are no changes in DAT-scan results in Alzheimer's disease compared to controls.

Walker Z *et al*. Dementia with Lewy bodies: a comparison of clinical diagnosis, FP-CIT single photon emission computed tomography imaging and autopsy. *Journal of Neurology, Neurosurgery and Psychiatry* 2007; **78**: 1176–1181.

70. A. Beta >13 Hz, Alpha 8 to 13 Hz, Theta 4 to 7Hz, Delta < 3Hz. In normal, awake adults lying quietly with the eyes closed, an 8- to 13-Hz alpha rhythm is seen over the occipital region, which is attenuated when the eyes are opened. During drowsiness, the alpha rhythm is again attenuated; with light sleep, slower activity in the theta (4 to 7 Hz) and delta (4 Hz) ranges becomes more apparent. A generalized, faster beta activity (13 Hz) is seen more anteriorly during active wakefulness. Beta activity may be prominent in patients receiving barbiturate or benzodiazepine drugs. Adults normally may show a small amount of theta activity over the temporal regions when awake. A disproportionate increase in slow wave activity should raise suspicions about cerebral pathology.

Bradley GW, *et al*., eds. *Neurology in Clinical Practice*, 4th edn. Butterworth-Heineman, 2003, pp. 465–491.

71. E. Slow triphasic waves are typically seen in metabolic encephalopathies such as hepatic failure. Hypsarrhythmia is associated with infantile spasms (West's syndrome). Three-Hz spike-and-wave activity associated with typical absence attacks. Generalized multiple spikes and waves (poly-spike wave) are associated with myoclonic epilepsy. In most cases of delirium, generalized slowing is noted. In delirium tremens and delirium due to withdrawal of sedatives, fast-frequency EEG may be obtained.

Bradley GW, *et al*., eds. *Neurology in Clinical Practice*, 4th edn. Butterworth-Heineman, 2003, pp. 465–491.

72. B. EEG during ECT treatment shows sharp waves and spikes during the seizure. This must be recorded equally well on both EEG electrode leads to be confident of a generalized seizure activity. Clearly observable cessation point and good postictal suppression (flattening) are other features aiding confirmation of ictal activity on electric stimulation. See-saw pattern in sleep EEG is noted during REM sleep.

Bradley GW, *et al*., eds. *Neurology in Clinical Practice*, 4th edn. Butterworth-Heineman, 2003, pp. 465–491.

73. C. A characteristic neurological feature associated with hypothyroidism is delayed relaxation of deep tendon reflexes. This produces a slow and sluggish reflex. Hypertonia occurs in upper motor neurone lesions. Clonus is a sign of extremely brisk deep tendon reflex, often demonstrated at the ankles. It is a pyramidal sign. Loss of deep tendon reflexes should raise suspicion of a lower motor neurone lesion, for example motor neuropathy. Exaggerated jaw jerk is seen in pseudobulbar palsy, which can occur in motor neurone diseases such as amyotrophic lateral sclerosis.

Garden G. Physical examination in psychiatric practice. *Advances in Psychiatric Treatment* 2005; **11**: 142–149.

74. C.   Insertion of cardiac pacemaker precludes MRI study as the magnetic field can disturb the pacemaker rhythm. Increased iron content, as in haemochromatosis, has no effect on MRI clinically! Due to the absence of exposure to radiation of X-ray frequency, pregnancy is not a contraindication to undergo MRI scanning. Patients with a significant degree of claustrophobia might experience intense anxiety while undergoing MRI scan within the closed space of a scanner as undergoing MRI scanning is a more time consuming process than a plain X ray. Learning disability or epilepsy *per se* are not contraindications for MRI.

Kasper DL, *et al.*, eds. *Harrison's Principles of Internal Medicine*, 16th edn. McGraw-Hill, 2005, p. 2350.

75. A.   Various guidelines exist for diagnosing dementia. Most of them endorse routinely using clinical interview, especially on the lines of the DSM Definition of Dementia, for making a diagnosis of dementia. To specify subtypes of dementia, guidelines from consortium for DLB, consensus criteria for FTD, consensus for CJD, or Hachinski ischaemic index for vascular dementia may be useful. Sophisticated imaging techniques are not necessary for clinical diagnosis of dementia, for example volumetric MRI or CT measurement strategies.

AGS Clinical Practice Committee. American Academy of Neurology's dementia guidelines for early detection, diagnosis, and management of dementia. *Journal of the American Geriatrics Society* 2003; **51**: 869.

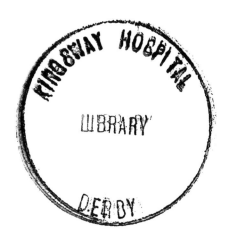

CORE CLINICAL PSYCHIATRY

1. **The majority of postpartum psychotic episodes are characterized by which of the following presentations?**
   A. Schizophreniform presentation
   B. Affective–manic presentation
   C. Delirium–organic presentation
   D. Dissociative presentation
   E. Catatonic presentation

2. **Which of the following figures represent the correct estimate of the incidence of postpartum psychosis?**
   A. Around 1–2 in 1000
   B. Around 1 in 100
   C. Around 1 in 10,000
   D. Around 5 in 100
   E. Around 1 in 2000

3. **Which of the following postpartum disorders is correctly matched with its time of onset?**
   A. Postpartum blues – within a few months of delivery
   B. Postpartum depression – first week of delivery
   C. Postpartum psychosis – within 2 weeks of delivery
   D. Postpartum pituitary apoplexy –12 months after delivery
   E. All of the above are correct

4. **Which of the following principle has guided the organization of disorders in ICD-10 Chapter V?**
   A. Hierarchy
   B. Reversibility
   C. Treatment response
   D. Mode of onset
   E. Degree of disability

5. **In ICD-10 schizoaffective disorder is included in the same chapter as which of the following disorders?**

    A. Schizophrenia
    B. Affective disorders
    C. Organic disorders
    D. Stress disorders
    E. Personality disorders

6. **Which of the following principles is not included in psychiatric classificatory systems (ICD and DSM) to define specific psychiatric disorders?**

    A. Number of symptoms
    B. Impairment criteria
    C. Duration criteria
    D. Prognostic criteria
    E. Exclusion criteria

7. **Which of the following is a difference between DSM-IV and ICD-10?**

    A. Culture-bound syndromes are separately classified in ICD
    B. Comorbid diagnoses are allowed in DSM
    C. DSM-IV has a dimensional approach to personality disorders
    D. Length of illness is a criteria for diagnosing DSM-IV schizophrenia
    E. Schizotypal disorder is a personality disorder in ICD-10

8. **In the multiaxial system of DSM-IV, the fifth axis refers to**

    A. General medical condition
    B. Personality difficulties
    C. Global assessment of functioning
    D. Psychosocial stress factors
    E. Intelligence level

9. **Two clinicians using the same checklist to aid clinical description come up with the same diagnosis. Which of the following properties of the checklist is involved in this outcome?**

    A. Validity of the checklist
    B. Reliability of checklist
    C. Sensitivity of checklist
    D. Specificity of checklist
    E. None of the above

10. **Which of the following could increase the validity of psychiatric diagnosis in the future?**

    A. Cross-cultural studies
    B. Laboratory tests
    C. Operational criteria
    D. Cross-sectional studies
    E. Consensus statements

11. **Which of the following is a benefit of a categorical classification over dimensional classification?**

    A. Easy to communicate
    B. Increased validity
    C. Prognostic information
    D. Informs qualitative research
    E. All of the above

12. **Which of the following disorders has the most evidence for existing as a continuum in the population, making a dimensional approach more rational?**

    A. Delusional disorders
    B. Personality disorders
    C. Developmental disorders
    D. Affective disorders
    E. Cognitive disorders

13. **By definition, the nature of delirium that differentiates it from dementia includes which of the following?**

    A. Insidious onset
    B. Acute onset
    C. Deteriorating course
    D. Familial onset
    E. Irreversible progression

14. **Which of the following best describes the nature of cognitive impairment required to diagnose dementia?**

    A. Focal, progressive deficits
    B. Focal, static deficits
    C. Global, progressive deficits
    D. Global, static deficits
    E. None of the above

15. **The most common cause of presenile dementia is**

    A. Vascular dementia
    B. Pick's dementia
    C. Alzheimer's dementia
    D. Lewy body dementia
    E. Prion dementia

16. **Which one of the following is NOT a risk factor for developing dementia?**

    A. Smoking
    B. Boxing
    C. Ageing
    D. Drinking alcohol
    E. Living alone

17. **The best option for preventing dementia available currently is**
    A. Regular NSAIDs
    B. Vitamin E
    C. Low salt diet
    D. Early retirement
    E. None of the above

18. **Which one of the following genetic factor is associated with senile dementia of Alzheimer's type?**
    A. Presenilin 1 only
    B. Presenilin 1 and 2
    C. Amyloid precursor protein
    D. *APOE4* allele
    E. Defective tau protein

19. **With respect to the major classificatory systems ICD and DSM, the term 'operational definition' refers to which of the following?**
    A. Definition arrived at by a consensus
    B. Definition with precise inclusion and exclusion criteria
    C. Definition validated by field trials
    D. Definition with strict duration of illness criteria
    E. Definitions with multilingual translation

20. **Dementia secondary to which of the following is not reversible?**
    A. Nutritional deficiencies
    B. Hypothyroidism
    C. Stroke
    D. Normal pressure hydrocephalus
    E. Depression

21. **Which of the following produce a rapidly evolving dementia with neurological features?**
    A. Viruses
    B. Prions
    C. Bacteria
    D. Helminths
    E. Drugs

22. **Prion dementia is caused by all of the following EXCEPT**
    A. Hormone extracts
    B. Corneal transplants
    C. Organ donations
    D. Peritoneal dialysis
    E. Contaminated meat

23. **The probability of developing Korsakoff's syndrome is related to which of the following features?**

A. Amount of alcohol consumed
B. Nutritional deprivation
C. Age of onset of drinking
D. Type of alcoholic drink
E. Level of tolerance

24. **Korsakoff's syndrome is characterized by all EXCEPT**

A. Dense anterograde amnesia
B. Impaired procedural memory
C. Apathy
D. Confabulation
E. Executive deficits

25. **Which of the following best describes the triad characteristic of normal pressure hydrocephalus?**

A. Ataxia, dementia, confabulation
B. Incontinence, dementia, confabulation
C. Headaches, visual disturbances, dementia
D. Headaches, ataxia, dementia
E. Ataxia, dementia, incontinence

26. **Which one of the following clinical signs and diseases is correctly paired?**

A. Wilson's disease–chorea
B. Huntington's disease–dystonia
C. Parkinson's disease–tremors
D. Pseudobulabr palsy–past pointing
E. Motor neuron disease–ataxia

27. **A 40-year-old man develops irritability and depressed mood with significant personality change. His father committed suicide at age of 45 and grandmother suffered from memory problems before she died at age 57. Which is the most important diagnosis to consider in this case?**

A. Parkinson's disease
B. Wilson's disease
C. Huntington's disease
D. Sydenham's chorea
E. Fahr's disease

28. **A 45-year-old man develops auditory hallucinations that are initially fragmented but later turns into second person derogatory. The most important aspect of personal history in this case is**

    A. Stimulant use
    B. Alcohol use
    C. Relationship difficulties
    D. Psychosexual history
    E. Employment history

29. **Mr Smith considers himself as an alcoholic. He uses the same brand of whisky everyday and drinks at the same pub around the same time. Which of the following features is he exhibiting?**

    A. Salience
    B. Tolerance
    C. Narrow repertoire
    D. Loss of control
    E. Relief drinking

30. **Which of the following clinical feature of schizophrenia adds support to a neurodevelopmental hypothesis?**

    A. Age of onset
    B. Stress-induced relapses
    C. Increased incidence among migrants
    D. Association with cannabis
    E. Response to antipsychotics

31. **A 32-year-old man presents to a dermatologist with circumscribed areas of alopecia. He admits to recurrent pulling of his hair, especially at times of stress. He feels a sense of relief after the act. He has a normal IQ and no other stereotyped behaviour. Which of the following is the most appropriate diagnosis?**

    A. OCD
    B. Tourette's syndrome
    C. Trichotillomania
    D. Autism
    E. Factitious disorder

32. **Risk of developing schizophrenia is increased in which of the following populations?**

    A. Learning disabled population
    B. Female sex
    C. Single parent families
    D. Sexually abused children
    E. Older mothers

33. **Which of the following is an important difference between male and female schizophrenia?**

    A. Males have later onset and better prognosis
    B. Males have earlier onset and better prognosis
    C. Females have later onset and poor prognosis
    D. Females have later onset and better prognosis
    E. Females have earlier onset and poor prognosis

34. **What is the risk of developing schizophrenia in a concordant monozygotic twin?**

    A. Less than 35%
    B. Around 45%
    C. Around 70%
    D. Around 12%
    E. Around 90%

35. **Which is a chromosomal deletion syndrome closely related to schizophrenia phenotype?**

    A. Edward's syndrome
    B. Patau syndrome
    C. di George syndrome
    D. Cri du Chat syndrome
    E. Laurence–Moon–Biedl syndrome

36. **A 20-year-old man repeatedly cross-dresses in privacy. He experiences sexual arousal during cross-dressing but has a normal sexual relationship with his girlfriend otherwise. Which of the following is the appropriate diagnosis?**

    A. Disorder of gender identity
    B. Disorder of sexual preference
    C. Disorder of sexual orientation
    D. Disorder of chromosomal sex
    E. Sexual dysfunction of arousal phase

37. **A 19-year-old boy shows recent onset avolition, flat affect, preoccupation with religion and philosophy. He preferred being solitary most of his childhood. Most probable diagnosis include**

    A. Simple schizophrenia
    B. Paranoid schizophrenia
    C. Hebephrenic schizophrenia
    D. Residual schizophrenia
    E. Schizoaffective disorder

38. **Which of the following with regard to cannabis use in schizophrenia is incorrect?**
    A. Cannabis use could be a self medication attempt
    B. Both schizophrenia and cannabis use are high in lower socioeconomic group
    C. Psychosis in cannabis users may be mediated by polymorphisms in COMT
    D. Cannabis is associated with schizophrenia in a dose-dependent fashion
    E. Cannabis intoxication is indistinguishable from schizophrenia

39. **A 38-year-old man had his most recent episode of schizophrenic relapse 6 months ago. Though he responded well to antipsychotics he still hears occasional voices. Currently he has lost sleep, appetite, and weight and complains of low energy and pervasive anhedonia with low mood. This description best fits which of the following diagnosis?**
    A. Schizoaffective disorder
    B. Psychotic depression
    C. Postschizophrenic depression
    D. Dysthymia
    E. Unremitted schizophrenia

40. **A 37-year-old lady has an eccentric hobby of preserving animal carcasses found on roadside. She also has suspiciousness, magical thinking, and obsessive ruminations though she does not resist them. She has never had a diagnosis of schizophrenia. This description best fits which of the following diagnosis?**
    A. Schizoid personality
    B. Schizotypal disorder
    C. Paranoid personality
    D. Obsessive compulsive disorder
    E. Simple schizophrenia

41. **How long does the natural course of an episode of untreated mania last?**
    A. 4 weeks
    B. 4 months
    C. 6 weeks
    D. 9 months
    E. 2 weeks

42. **Which of the following is NOT a part of ICD-10 somatic syndrome of depression?**
    A. Loss of appetite
    B. Loss of libido
    C. Loss of sleep
    D. Constipation
    E. Loss of energy

43. A 32-year-old lady is incapacitated by recurrent panic attacks. She feels low and cannot leave her home, leading to loss of interest in leisure activities. She feels guilty for not being a good mother for her 12-year-old son as she finds routine housework extremely demanding. This description best fits which of the following diagnosis?

   A. Depressive disorder
   B. Agoraphobia
   C. Panic disorder
   D. Generalized anxiety disorder
   E. Chronic fatigue syndrome

44. Which of the following is incorrect with regard to social phobia?

   A. Younger age of onset than other phobias
   B. Symptoms more pronounced in large groups
   C. Blushing is more common than in other anxiety disorders
   D. Fear of vomiting in public may be seen
   E. Marked avoidance behaviour is noted

45. Which of the following is the endocrine abnormality most commonly seen in depression?

   A. Hypercortisolaemia
   B. Hypocortisolaemia
   C. Hypothyroidism
   D. Hypopituitarism
   E. Hypoprolactinaemia

46. Which of the following is noted through longitudinal observation of recurrent depressive disorder?

   A. Life events precede onset of each relapse
   B. Life events are more common in later episodes
   C. Life events are more common in earlier than later episodes
   D. No relationship is noted between life events and relapses
   E. Life events precede only the first episode

47. Which of the following endocrine abnormalities is suspected to be associated with rapid cycling bipolar disorder?

   A. Hypercortisolaemia
   B. Hypocortisolaemia
   C. Hypothyroidism
   D. Hypopituitarism
   E. Hyperprolactinaemia

48. **Which of the following is NOT a predictor of good outcome in schizophrenia?**

    A. Florid positive symptoms at onset
    B. Prominent affective symptoms
    C. Acute onset
    D. Older age of onset
    E. Long first episode

49. **Which of the following is NOT a characteristic feature of atypical depression?**

    A. Leaden paralysis
    B. Reversed vegetative signs
    C. Response to MAO inhibitors
    D. Rejection sensitivity
    E. Obsessional symptoms

50. **Which of the following is a good estimate of heritability of bipolar disorder?**

    A. 10%
    B. 25%
    C. 80%
    D. 40%
    E. 95%

51. **Even a single episode of mania warrants a diagnosis of bipolar disorder in DSM-IV. What is the proportion of patients with pure recurrent mania without depression among these patients?**

    A. 20%
    B. 10%
    C. 5%
    D. 30%
    E. 40%

52. **A patient with a family history of affective disorders presents with recurrent periods of elated mood and grandiose delusions believing that he is King Solomon. These episodes last for only 4 days. Which of the following is the most appropriate diagnosis?**

    A. Bipolar disorder type 1
    B. Bipolar disorder type 2
    C. Mixed affective state
    D. Cyclothymia
    E. None of the above

53. **Which of the following is the most important diagnostic information that differentiates bipolar disorder from schizophrenia?**
    A. Interepisode recovery
    B. Presence of delusions
    C. Religious content of hallucinations
    D. Family history
    E. History of cannabis use

54. **Which of the following statements about the gender distribution of affective disorders is correct?**
    A. Bipolar incidence is equal in both sexes
    B. Unipolar depression is more common in men
    C. Age of onset differs with gender
    D. In childhood, girls are more depressed than boys
    E. Rapid cycling is more common in men

55. **According to twin studies, the strongest evidence of a genetic cause is for which of the following disorders?**
    A. Schizophrenia
    B. Bipolar disorder
    C. Unipolar depression
    D. Conduct disorder
    E. Alcohol – harmful use

56. **To diagnose 'double depression' the patient must have a primary diagnosis of which of the following disorders?**
    A. Recurrent depressive disorder
    B. Cyclothymia
    C. Dysthymia
    D. Brief recurrent depression
    E. Alcohol dependence

57. **Which of the following is a medical condition in which symptoms similar to OCD are found?**
    A. Sydenham's chorea
    B. Guillain–Barré syndrome
    C. Motor neurone disease
    D. Hashimoto's thyroiditis
    E. Cystic fibrosis

58. **Strong risk factors for depression include all of the following EXCEPT**
    A. Neuroticism
    B. Life events
    C. Past history of depression
    D. Low IQ
    E. Family history

59. Which of the following is true regarding the clinical presentation of OCD?

A. Acute onset

B. Early presentation to clinic

C. Long duration of untreated illness

D. Chronic deteriorating course

E. All of the above

60. A 17-year-old patient has recurrent intrusive thoughts which he perceives to be senseless and involuntary. He starts believing these thoughts are being inserted by his family members though these are his own thoughts. Which of the following diagnoses must be considered apart from OCD?

A. Schizophrenia

B. Anankastic personality

C. Depression

D. Schizotypal disorder

E. Delusional disorder

61. A 12-year-old boy repeatedly wakes up in middle of night screaming, but could recall only fragments of any mental images. He appears to be disoriented for several minutes on waking. Which of the following diagnoses is the most appropriate?

A. Nightmares

B. Night terrors

C. Sleep apnoea

D. Narcolepsy

E. REM sleep behavioural disorder

62. A 25-year-old man has had irrational fear for darkness since childhood. He is not distressed about this currently and does not take special measures to avoid being in the dark. Which of the following is true?

A. He has a specific phobia as he has an irrational fear

B. He has a specific phobia as he has had it since childhood

C. He has no specific phobia as he does not have avoidance behaviour

D. He has no specific phobia as fear of darkness is common

E. He has a specific phobia with loss of insight

63. Which one of the following specific phobias is strongly genetic?

A. Animal phobia

B. Space phobia

C. Blood injury injection phobia

D. Acrophobia

E. Spider phobia

64. **Which one of the following features during trauma has the capacity to predict future development of PTSD?**

    A. Anterograde amnesia immediately after trauma
    B. Emotional numbing during trauma
    C. Panic attack during trauma
    D. Crying during trauma
    E. Autonomic arousal during trauma

65. **Which of the following is NOT a feature of panic disorder?**

    A. Situational panic attacks
    B. Situationally predisposed attacks
    C. Out of the blue panic attacks
    D. Nocturnal panic attacks
    E. Unilateral panic attack

66. **Which of the following is an early developmental temperament noted to precede the onset of social phobia in some cases?**

    A. Behavioural familiarity
    B. Behavioural stimulation
    C. Behavioural inhibition
    D. Temper tantrums
    E. Cognitive inhibition

67. **Which of the following describes the two peaks often noted in the age distribution of panic disorder?**

    A. Around age 20 and 50
    B. Around age 30 and 50
    C. Around age 20 and 40
    D. Around age 30 and 40
    E. Around age 50 and 70

68. **Which one of the following suggests depression rather than a grief reaction?**

    A. Early morning awakening
    B. Blaming oneself for the death
    C. Complaining of symptoms suffered by the dead person
    D. Suicidal ideas
    E. Preoccupation with the death

69. **According to Brown and Harris, all of the following predispose to depression following a stressful life event EXCEPT**

    A. Early parental loss
    B. Unemployment
    C. Parental responsibility
    D. Lack of confidant
    E. Living in rural isolation

70. **A woman suffers from recurrent, intrusive flashbacks of a fire accident that she had in the past, accompanied by irritability and sleeplessness. In order to diagnose PTSD, when should the fire accident have happened?**

    A. Within the last 6 months
    B. Within the last 9 months
    C. Within the last 12 months
    D. Within the last 18 months
    E. Within the last 4 weeks

71. **Which one of the following is NOT a poor prognostic factor in OCD?**

    A. Male gender
    B. Poor insight
    C. Early onset
    D. Family history of OCD
    E. Presence of depressive symptoms

72. **Which of the following is the most common method of attempting self harm in UK?**

    A. Paracetamol overdose
    B. Benzodiazepine overdose
    C. Hanging
    D. Car exhaust
    E. Jumping from heights

73. **What is the proportion of suicide victims who attended their primary care practitioner within 4 weeks prior to suicide?**

    A. 33%
    B. 25%
    C. 66%
    D. 40%
    E. 13%

74. **A patient has tenacious sense of personal rights, leading on to repeated quarrels with neighbours. A personality disorder to be considered is**

    A. Anankastic PD
    B. Dependent PD
    C. Passive aggressive PD
    D. Paranoid PD
    E. Borderline PD

75. **Which of the following is feature of schizoid personality disorder?**

    A. Inability to plan ahead
    B. Sensitivity to rejection
    C. Indifference to praise or criticism
    D. Excessive self importance
    E. Impulsivity and lack of self restraint

76. Excessive concern with physical appearance, shallow, labile affect, and egocentricity are a feature of which of the following?
    A. Histrionic personality
    B. Narcissistic personality
    C. Antisocial personality
    D. Borderline personality
    E. Dysmorphophobia

77. Fear of abandonment is a feature of borderline personality. It is also seen in which other personality disorder?
    A. Avoidant personality
    B. Dependent personality
    C. Histrionic personality
    D. Anankastic personality
    E. None of the above

78. Which personality disorder is considered to be closely associated with bipolar diathesis?
    A. Borderline personality
    B. Narcissistic personality
    C. Antisocial personality
    D. Schizoid personality
    E. Schizotypal personality

79. Which is the most common major mental illness in patients with anankastic personality?
    A. OCD
    B. Schizophrenia
    C. Depression
    D. Generalized anxiety disorder
    E. Eating disorder

80. The percentage of schizophrenic patients who ultimately commit suicide is approximately
    A. 1%
    B. 5%
    C. 10%
    D. 20%
    E. 30%

81. What is the estimated risk of developing schizophrenia throughout the lifetime of an average person in the population?
    A. 1 in 150
    B. 1 in 1000
    C. 1 in 500
    D. 1 in 100
    E. 1 in 30

82. **Which of the following is NOT true with respect to narcolepsy?**

   A. Sleep onset REM
   B. Abnormalities in routine EEG
   C. HLA-DR2 associated
   D. Sleep paralysis is seen
   E. Autosomal dominant inheritance is noted

83. **Somnambulism is a disorder of which stage of sleep?**

   A. REM
   B. Slow wave
   C. Stage 2 NREM
   D. Stage 1 NREM
   E. Any of the above

84. **Which of the following is a sleep disturbance characteristic of mania?**

   A. Reduced early morning sleep
   B. Reduced initial sleep
   C. Reduced need for sleep
   D. Reduced latency of sleep
   E. None of the above

85. **Which of the following is NOT a medical cause of panic attacks?**

   A. Hypoglycaemia
   B. Arrythmias
   C. Mitral valve prolapse syndrome
   D. Hypothyroidism
   E. Phaeochromocytoma

86. **Which of the following statements with respect to the natural history of eating disorders is true?**

   A. Nearly 50% of patients with bulimia have a past history of anorexia nervosa.
   B. Nearly 50% of patients with anorexia nervosa have a past history of bulimia.
   C. Bulimia and anorexia nervosa coexist simultaneously in 50% of patients.
   D. Bulimia and anorexia are mutually exclusive diagnoses.
   E. 80% of anorexia patients achieve complete remission in 6 months.

87. **Dementia can be differentiated from pseudodementia by all of the following EXCEPT**

   A. Verbal memory
   B. Visuospatial function
   C. Executive functions
   D. Motor disturbances
   E. Frontal release signs

88. **Which one of the following statement about paraphrenia is NOT correct? Paraphrenia is**

    A. Common in females
    B. Often associated with sensory impairment
    C. Associated with premorbid paranoid personality
    D. Associated with prominent negative symptoms
    E. Associated with persecutory delusions

89. **Multiple personality disorder is a controversial diagnosis described under which of the following group of disorders?**

    A. Personality disorders
    B. Organic disorders
    C. Schizophrenia
    D. Dissociative disorders
    E. Not included in either DSM-IV or ICD-10

90. **Which of the following symptoms is/are a characteristic feature in dissociative fugue?**

    A. Depressive symptoms
    B. Depersonalization symptoms
    C. Defective new learning
    D. Wandering far away with assumption of a new identity
    E. Family history of epilepsy

91. **Which of the following is a feature of chronic fatigue syndrome?**

    A. Disproportionate fatigue compared to exertion
    B. Fatigue is not relieved by adequate rest
    C. Fatigue is of new onset
    D. Joint aches and tender points are noted
    E. All of the above

92. **Which of the following best differentiates hypochondriasis from somatoform disorder?**

    A. Patients with hypochondriasis are concerned about symptoms rather than diagnosis
    B. Hypochondriacal patients ask for treatment rather than investigations
    C. Somatizing patients are concerned about diagnosis
    D. Somatizing patients ask for treatment and symptom relief
    E. Hypochondriasis responds better to treatment

93. **A young lady develops transient bladder incontinence coinciding with a recent job loss. A few months later she presents to her GP with weakness of the right leg. Which of the following medical disorder is often confused with conversion disorder?**
    A. Myasthenia gravis
    B. Guillain-Barré syndrome
    C. Brain tumour
    D. Creutzfeldt–Jakob disease
    E. Multiple sclerosis

94. **Which of the following is the single most important factor predicting suicide risk?**
    A. Recent life event
    B. Family history of suicide
    C. Past history of suicidal attempt
    D. Recent discharge from hospital
    E. None of the above

95. **You are bleeped to assess five patients at the same time at A & E. Which one of the following has highest risk of suicide compared to the others?**
    A. 32-year-old woman with obsessional symptoms
    B. 56-year-old widower who tried to gas himself using an exhaust
    C. 22-year-old girl presenting after a recent break-up, having consumed alcohol before calling her boy friend and taking an overdose
    D. 83-year-old cognitively impaired lady who took eight instead of four sleeping pills on the same day of prescription
    E. 41-year-old heroin user demanding methadone from A & E

96. **Prevalence of major depression among patients with dementia is**
    A. 10%
    B. 50%
    C. 15%
    D. 20%
    E. 35%

97. **A 45-year-old man presents to A & E with complaints of hearing voices. On further questioning he claims amnesia for the content of these voices and reveals he has lost his tenancy the previous day due to aggressive behaviour. An important diagnosis to consider is**
    A. Malingering
    B. Depression
    C. Temporal lobe epilepsy
    D. Factitious disorder
    E. Stress reaction

98. **A 16-year-old boy presents with cycles of sleepiness lasting for weeks associated with excessive weight gain and hunger. Which of the following is an appropriate diagnosis?**

   A. Stein Leventhal syndrome
   B. Klein–Levine syndrome
   C. Klüver–Bucy syndrome
   D. Dorian Gray syndrome
   E. Charles Bonnet syndrome

99. **Which one of the following sleep disturbances is associated with Parkinson's disease?**

   A. Somnambulism
   B. Sleep talking
   C. Night terrors
   D. REM behavioural disorder
   E. Sleep bruxism

100. **A 32-year-old man presents with beliefs that he has a chip in his brain that could neutralize all nuclear radiations in his presence. He stops often in mid sentence and continues conversation on a different theme altogether. Which of the following neurological conditions mimics thought blocking?**

   A. Multiple sclerosis
   B. Infantile seizures
   C. Absence seizures
   D. Atonic seizures
   E. Narcolepsy

1. B. It is well known that postpartum psychosis is often an episode of bipolar manic illness. A small minority have schizophreniform presentation or organic, delirious presentation. Another episode of relapse occurs in the same year in nearly 70% and risk during subsequent pregnancy is greater than 50%. In delirious presentations, ruling out organic cause, such as postpartum pituitary apoplexy, is very important.

Sadock BJ and Sadock VA. *Kaplan & Sadock's Synopsis of Psychiatry: Behavioral Sciences/Clinical Psychiatry*, 10th edn. Lippincott Williams & Wilkins, 2007, p. 866.

2. A. Postpartum psychosis affects 1 to 2 per 1000 childbirths. Initially, it was claimed that the incidence was higher in the West but, currently, comparable rates have been obtained worldwide. In contrast, postpartum depression affects 10 to 15% of all mothers, while postpartum blues affects 50 to 70% of mothers.

Sadock BJ and Sadock VA. *Kaplan & Sadock's Synopsis of Psychiatry: Behavioral Sciences/Clinical Psychiatry*, 10th edn. Lippincott Williams & Wilkins, 2007, p. 866.
Also see
Johnstone EC *et al.*, eds. *Companion to Psychiatric Studies*, 7th edn. Churchill Livingstone, 2004, p. 747.

3. C. Time of onset of symptoms is an important clue in postpartum illnesses, especially to aid diagnosis during early presentation. Postpartum blues typically start 3 to 5 days after delivery; postpartum psychosis is also of acute onset and can develop between 2 weeks and 2 months after delivery; postpartum depression can occur anytime between 2 months and 1 year after childbirth, most commonly in the third month.

Sadock BJ and Sadock VA. *Kaplan & Sadock's Synopsis of Psychiatry: Behavioral Sciences/Clinical Psychiatry*, 10th edn. Lippincott Williams & Wilkins, 2007, p. 867.

4. A. Jasperian hierarchy refers to the principle that, in psychiatric practice, some diagnoses when made preclude using another diagnostic label even if a second diagnosis could account for a constellation of symptoms. For example when a diagnosis of major depression is made, symptoms of generalized anxiety are included in the description of depression itself; a separate diagnosis of generalized anxiety disorder need not be entertained. Similarly, depressive symptoms can be present during an acute psychotic episode of schizophrenia – they need not always indicate a separate diagnosis of depression. The hierarchy is maintained in ICD-10, to some extent, in the way the various chapters of ICD are organized. Organic disorders trump a diagnosis of psychotic disorders, which in turn are more or less equally considered with affective disorders. Affective disorders trump neuroses, which in turn trump personality disorders. DSM has abandoned this hierarchy to a large extent, though the principle is retained. Different modes of onset or degrees of disability will not yield differing diagnosis. Treatment response cannot be considered as a principle for organization of ICD-10 Chapter V.

Johnstone EC *et al.*, eds. *Companion to Psychiatric Studies*, 7th edn. Churchill Livingstone, 2004, p. 247.

5. A.   Schizoaffective disorder is a diagnosis that lies between schizophrenia and affective disorder. It is placed together with schizophrenia in section F20–29. ICD-10 stipulates that schizophrenic and affective symptoms must be simultaneously present and both must be equally prominent. In DSM-IV the concept of a continuum between psychosis and affective illness is better highlighted. According to DSM-IV: (1) both schizophrenia and affective disorder categories must be met simultaneously; (2) a period of psychosis (2 weeks) without prominent affective symptoms must be present; and (3) the mood disturbance must be present for a substantial period during active (psychotic) and residual periods. Note that in postschizophrenic depression (classified under schizophrenia in ICD-10) the psychotic symptoms must not be prominent (but residual) when a depressive episode is present, and depression must be within 12 months of the most recent psychotic episode. Schizophreniform disorder is a diagnosis used when schizophrenia does not fulfil the duration criteria in DSM-IV (<6 months). This diagnosis is not included in ICD-10.

World Health Organization. *The ICD-10 Classification of Mental and Behavioral Disorders; Clinical Descriptions and Diagnostic Guidelines.* Geneva: World Health Organization, 1992, p. 106.

6. D.   In general, both DSM and ICD use symptom count, age of onset, duration, impairment, and exclusion criteria for many psychiatric diagnoses. Aetiological information and theoretical speculations are avoided in classification. Course specifiers are used often in DSM-IV to aid in subtyping a disorder. Good or poor prognostic typology is not employed as a classification principle in either of these systems.

Semple DM *et al.*, eds. *Oxford Handbook of Psychiatry*, 1st edn. Oxford University Press, 2005, pp. 8, 9.

7. D.   In DSM-IV a period of at least 6 months of observation is required before a reliable diagnosis of schizophrenia could be made. In ICD-10 a period of 1 month is used instead. This makes DSM-IV schizophrenia narrower than ICD-10 schizophrenia. Schizotypal disorder is a personality disorder according to DSM-IV not ICD-10. Culture-bound syndromes are separately coded in DSM, which is largely an American system. ICD-10 encompasses cultural differences in various places throughout the text.

World Health Organization. *The ICD-10 Classification of Mental and Behavioral Disorders; Clinical Descriptions and Diagnostic Guidelines.* Geneva: World Health Organization, 1992, p. 86.

8. C.   DSM is multiaxial – it consists of five axes:

Axis 1. Primary psychiatric diagnosis
Axis 2. Personality difficulties or learning difficulties; can include defence mechanism/ coping strategy employed predominantly
Axis 3. General medical condition (may or may not be related to Axis 1 or 2)
Axis 4. Psychosocial stressor (both positive and negative)
Axis 5. Global assessment of functioning (highest score achieved over a few months in the last year in various domains of life)

Note that ICD-10 also has a multiaxial version, which has three axes.

Sadock BJ and Sadock VA. *Kaplan & Sadock's Synopsis of Psychiatry: Behavioral Sciences/Clinical Psychiatry*, 10th edn. Lippincott Williams & Wilkins, 2007, p. 306.

9. B. Reliability of a test refers to its ability to produce the same results when tested at different times (test–retest reliability) or tested by different observers at the same time (observer reliability). Validity refers to the ability of a test to measure what it sets out or intends to measure. Sensitivity refers to the ability of a test to pick the highest number of true patients from a sample to whom it is administered. Specificity refers to the ability to identify the correct diagnosis among various different possibilities. Reliability of diagnostic classifications is enhanced by using operationalized check lists. Field trials enhance the validity. Reliability and validity need not always correlate. It is possible for many clinicians to make the same diagnosis which is not really right (reliable but invalid). Validity has a ceiling set by reliability – very low reliability can reduce validity though *vice versa* is not true.

Johnstone EC et al., eds. *Companion to Psychiatric Studies*, 7th edn. Churchill Livingstone, 2004, p. 253.

10. B. How can we know whether the diagnosis we make using a set of descriptions and observation is the true condition that a patient has? Cross-sectional studies of even a huge number of patients cannot answer this question. Longitudinal study of the patient in question can improve claims about a diagnosis – but classification systems are typically constructed to enable a clinician to make a diagnosis after a time-sliced, cross-sectional interview rather than a lifelong observation. We can ensure that everyone makes the same diagnosis by having a consensus statement or cross-cultural studies. Definite laboratory measures that are objective can, if developed, increase the validity of a diagnosis.

Johnstone EC et al., eds. *Companion to Psychiatric Studies*, 7th edn. Churchill Livingstone, 2004, p. 253.

11. A. Categorical classification refers to the current ICD-10 and DSM-IV approach of using mutually exclusive labels for diagnosis in an 'all or none' fashion. A diagnosis is either present or absent according to this system, very similar to the medical model – pneumonia is either present or absent. Relative advantages of a categorical system are (1) it is very familiar and not complex to construct; (2) it is easy to remember and communicate; and (3) it informs management decisions readily (e.g. if there is malaria, give chloroquine). A dimensional approach considers a continuum of diagnostic issues; it uses degrees of severity of a particular dimension (say mood, anxiety) rather than mutually exclusive 'boxes' of diagnosis. In this way various dimensions can be employed simultaneously to describe a patient's difficulties. Relative advantages of a dimensional system include: (1) more information is conveyed and this may include valuable information of prognostic importance that can be missed using plain categories; (2) it is very flexible; (3) it does not impose strict, artificial boundaries between disorders and so has better validity; and (4) it is more holistic and less labelling, thus informing qualitative research.

Johnstone EC et al., eds. *Companion to Psychiatric Studies*, 7th edn. Churchill Livingstone, 2004, p. 254.

12. B. It has been argued that personality disorders are better considered in a continuum with normalcy and so a dimensional approach is tipped for personality disorders in future DSM classifications. Note that contemporary cognitive psychologists consider delusions to exist in a continuum of normal beliefs and so a modular approach is criticized. But this does not imply that delusional disorders, as defined currently, exist in such a continuum.

Johnstone EC et al., eds. *Companion to Psychiatric Studies*, 7th edn. Churchill Livingstone, 2004, p. 254.

13. B. Delirium is an acute confusional state by definition. It may or may not be reversible depending on the aetiology. Most cases are reversible and have a non-deteriorating episodic course. Both dementia and delirium have an impact on global cognitive abilities, including memory.

World Health Organization. *The ICD-10 Classification of Mental and Behavioral Disorders; Clinical Descriptions and Diagnostic Guidelines*. Geneva: World Health Organization, 1992, p. 57.

14. C. Dementia is an organic syndrome wherein progressive, global cognitive disturbance is noted. Dementia is often irreversible. Cognitive disturbances include memory difficulties (amnesia), aphasia, agnosia, apraxia, impaired executive function, and personality changes. Significant psychosocial impairment must be present to warrant a diagnosis of dementia. Clouding of consciousness, impaired attention, wide diurnal fluctuation, presence of autonomic signs, and a high degree of reversibility on treating the potential cause are other differentiating features that point towards delirium.

Semple DM *et al.*, eds. *Oxford Handbook of Psychiatry*, 1st edn. Oxford University Press, 2005, p. 132.

15. C. Alzheimer's dementia is the most common dementia in both older and younger patients. Risk of Alzheimer's increases with age. About 1% risk at age 60 years then doubles every 5 years becoming nearly 40% of those aged 85 years. Women are affected three times more often. Down's syndrome, previous head injury, hypothyroidism, family history of dementia, and supposedly low educational attainment are other risk factors. Alzheimer's is implicated in up to two-thirds of all senile dementia.

Sampson EL *et al.* Young onset dementia. *Postgraduate Medical Journal* 2004; **80**: 125–139.

16. E. Smoking is a risk factor for dementia especially of the vascular type, though controversies exist as to whether smoking could prevent Alzheimer's disease. A large survey of UK male doctors followed up from 1951 has demonstrated that smoking in fact increases the risk of Alzheimer's. Also in a prospective, population-based cohort study of 6868 participants >55 years followed up for an average of 7 years, smoking was associated with increased risk of any dementia in general, and Alzheimer's in particular. Ageing increases the risk of dementia. Boxing is associated with dementia pugilistica wherein neurofibrillary tangles are observed. Alcoholic dementia occurs in excessive drinkers. Living alone does not increase the risk of dementia.

Reitz C *et al.* Relation between smoking and risk of dementia and Alzheimer disease: the Rotterdam Study. *Neurology* 2007; **69**: 998–1005.

17. E. Evidence for dementia preventive strategies has emerged recently though this is largely concerned with delaying the onset rather than abolishing the risk. Sustained use of NSAIDs is associated with a reduced risk of developing AD. Some NSAIDs appear to modulate the amyloid load in the brain. But NSAIDs have significant adverse effects that might limit their potential as primary preventive agents in AD. Oestrogens and HRT cannot be recommended and the potential of statins remains to be fully assessed. Evidence for using antioxidant supplements such as vitamin E and vitamin C is far from clear cut and there are safety concerns about higher doses of vitamin E. Strategies to target mid-life vascular risk factors are likely to have an important effect on the age of presentation of AD, though as of now none of the given options are recommended to prevent dementia.

Jones RW. Primary prevention of dementia. *Psychiatry* 2007; **6**: 511–513.

18. D. Of patients with Alzheimer's, 40% have a positive family history of Alzheimer's. This is especially true if the patient is younger (<55). Among various genes implicated, Chromosome 21 carries the gene for amyloid precursor protein (APP) which when mutant increases amyloid deposition even before senility, so it is associated with younger-onset dementia. Trisomy 21 acts via the same mechanism in Down's. The *APO* gene on chromosome 19 codes for apolipoprotein (apo). People with one copy of the *APOE4* allele have Alzheimer's three times more frequently than do those with no *APOE4* allele, and people with two *APOE4* alleles have the disease eight times more frequently. Diagnostic testing for *APOE4* is not recommended because it is seen in more patients without Alzheimer's than those with the disease and so accounts only for 50% of genetic variance. E3 is the most common *APOE* allele and E2 may be protective. It is possible that apoE4 mediates Alzheimer's risk via lipid metabolism as the presence of apoE4 increases cholesterol levels in blood. Chromosome 14 (presenilin 1) and chromosome 1 (presenilin 2) are also implicated in early-onset Alzheimer's via increased beta amyloid deposition.

Gelder MG *et al.*, eds. *New Oxford Textbook of Psychiatry*. Oxford University Press, 2000, p. 392.

19. B. The term operational definition refers to a definition that is specified by a series of precise, unambiguous inclusion and exclusion criteria. In other words, an operational definition is arrived at by using a checklist. This improves the reliability of a classificatory system tremendously. Before the popular use of ICD and DSM systems, the cross-national agreement for psychiatric diagnosis was very poor, as exemplified by the US–UK diagnostic study. In the UK, the rate of manic depression was ten times higher and the rate of schizophrenia was two times lower than the prevalence in the US (Cooper, 1972). Operational definitions paved the way for the wider use of standardized diagnostic instruments, increasing the reliability of classification.

Gelder MG *et al.*, ed. *Shorter Oxford Textbook of Psychiatry*, 5th edn. Oxford University Press, 2006, p. 30

Cooper JE. *et al. Psychiatric Diagnosis in New York and London*. Maudsley Monograph 20. Oxford: Oxford University Press, 1972.

20. C. Reversible causes constitute nearly 15% of initial diagnoses of dementia. The proportion is higher in younger patients. The reversible causes are commonly subdural haematoma, normal pressure hydrocephalus (NPH), vitamin B_{12} deficiency, metabolic causes, and hypothyroidism. Stroke causes vascular dementia which is irreversible.

Semple DM *et al.*, eds. *Oxford Handbook of Psychiatry*, 1st edn. Oxford University Press, 2005, p. 132.

21. B. Creutzfeldt–Jakob disease (CJD) is a prion disease that presents with rapidly evolving dementia with multiple neurological features. Prions are virus-like transmissible agents but without any nucleic acid. They are simple, mutated proteins originating from the normal human prion protein gene (*PRNP*), which is located on the short arm of chromosome 20. When mutant PrP^{Sc} is formed it is partially protease-resistant with a capacity to change further normal PrP to $PrP^{Sc,}$ initiating a cascade. CJD presents non-specifically with fatigue and flu-like symptoms with rapid development of neurological findings such as aphasia, cerebellar signs, myoclonus, apraxia with emotional lability, depression, delusions, hallucinations, or marked personality changes. The disease is rapidly progressive with dementia, akinetic mutism, coma, and death occurring within few months of onset.

Johnstone EC *et al.*, eds. *Companion to Psychiatric Studies*, 7th edn. Churchill Livingstone, 2004, p. 76.

22. D. Sporadic onset accounts for 85% of cases with CJD, while 10% result from genetic mutation. The remaining 5% result from iatrogenic transmission during transplant surgery of dura and corneal grafts, and pituitary growth hormone. vCJD is a variant form of human CJD that is transmitted by eating contaminated meat of an animal with bovine spongiform encephalopathy. Peritoneal dialysis does not involve foreign tissue.

Johnstone EC *et al.*, eds. *Companion to Psychiatric Studies*, 7th edn. Churchill Livingstone, 2004, p. 77.

23. B. Wernicke–Korsakoff syndrome is considered to be a nutritional illness seen in alcoholics. Thiamine deficiency can occur secondary to gastrectomy, carcinoma stomach, anorexia, haemodialysis, hyperemesis gravidarum, prolonged intravenous hyperalimentation, and alcoholism. This produces neuronal damage with small vessel hyperplasia and occasional haemorrhages especially in diencephalic structures such as mamillary bodies and medial dorsal thalamus. There is no clear correlation between amount, type, or duration of alcohol consumption and incidence of Korsakoff's syndrome. It is thought that patients who develop Korsakoff's may have abnormal transketolase enzyme, involved in thiamine metabolism.

Lishman WA. *Organic Psychiatry: The Psychological Consequences of Cerebral Disorder*, 3rd edn. Blackwell Science, 1997, p. 576.

24. B. In Korsakoff's syndrome recent memory tends to be affected more than is remote memory. Confabulation, apathy, and executive dysfunction are prominent. The length of retrograde amnesia is variable. Working memory and attention are preserved. The implicit emotional learning and procedural memory are preserved, facilitating rehabilitation; 75% of these patients show some degrees of improvement, whilst 25% show no change.

Semple DM *et al.*, eds. *Oxford Handbook of Psychiatry*, 1st edn. Oxford University Press, 2005, p. 530.

25. E. Normal pressure hydrocephalus or NPH is a syndrome of cerebral ventricular dilatation with normal CSF pressure. The changes are prominent in the third ventricle, affecting the pyramidal tract representing legs. This leads to a triad of: dementia, gait ataxia, and urinary incontinence. The dementia is reversible if NPH is treated promptly with shunt or repeated lumbar puncture.

Semple DM *et al.*, eds. *Oxford Handbook of Psychiatry*, 1st edn. Oxford University Press, 2005, p. 150.

26. C. In Wilson's disease athetosis with wing beating movements are noted. Huntington's disease is characterized by chorea while a patient with pseudobulbar palsy shows exaggerated jaw jerk and emotional lability. In motor neurone disease combined upper and lower motor neurone signs are noted. Ataxia typically occurs in posterior column, cerebellar, or vestibular damage. The tremor in Parkinson's is described as pill rolling tremor.

Semple DM *et al.*, eds. *Oxford Handbook of Psychiatry*, 1st edn. Oxford University Press, 2005, p. 170.

27. C. The clues in this case are young age of onset, presence of irritability, and personality change with family history including a degree of 'anticipation' over generations. Premature death, suicide, and psychiatric problems point to Huntington's disease in family members. The onset is usually during the fourth decade with significant numbers showing juvenile presentation with successive generations. The course is almost always a deteriorating pattern with death occurring around 10–12 years after diagnosis. Fahr's disease refers to idiopathic bilateral basal ganglia calcification.

Semple DM *et al.*, eds. *Oxford Handbook of Psychiatry*, 1st edn. Oxford University Press, 2005, p. 172.

28. B.   In alcoholic hallucinosis, psychotic symptoms start either during intoxication or withdrawal, but in a clear sensorium. The most common symptoms are auditory hallucinations; these are usually unstructured voices which can develop into persecutory or derogatory content. The hallucinations usually last for a short period and any persistence beyond 6 months is a strong suspicion for other psychotic illnesses such as schizophrenia.

Sadock BJ and Sadock VA. *Kaplan & Sadock's Synopsis of Psychiatry: Behavioral Sciences/Clinical Psychiatry*, 10th edn. Lippincott Williams & Wilkins, 2007, p. 400.

29. C.   Narrowed repertoire of drinking was included as one of the criteria for alcohol dependence by Griffith Edwards and Milton Gross in 1976. Heavy drinkers may have a wide drinking repertoire. This narrows as dependence advances. The dependent person may start to drink in a restricted pattern and manner every day, which would ensure a constant blood-alcohol level avoiding any symptoms of alcohol withdrawal. This is different from salience wherein priority is given to alcohol over other important areas of life and even painful consequences are disregarded.

Gelder MG *et al.*, eds. *New Oxford Textbook of Psychiatry*. Oxford University Press, 2000, p. 483.

30. A.   The peak ages of onset are 10 to 25 years for men and 25 to 35 years for women. Age of onset of schizophrenia is quoted as a supporting feature of neurodevelopmental hypothesis. A substantial reorganization of cortical connections, involving a programmed synaptic pruning, takes place during adolescence in humans. An excessive pruning of the prefrontal synapses, perhaps involving the excitatory glutamatergic inputs to pyramidal neurones, may underlie schizophrenia. This is called the Feinberg hypothesis.

Keshavan MS *et al.* Is schizophrenia due to excessive synaptic pruning in the prefrontal cortex? The Feinberg hypothesis revisited. *Journal of Psychiatric Research* 1994; **28**: 239–265.

31. C.   Stereotyped and recurrent pulling of hair with exacerbations during times of stress is characteristic of an impulse control disorder called trichotillomania. Similar to other impulse control disorders such as kleptomania, there is a sense of relief associated with the act. This commonly involves the scalp, facial hair, or axillary hair. The prognosis in children is better than adults; the latter often show a chronic fluctuating course. Some patients may bite the pulled hair, and complications such as intestinal obstruction can occur, especially in children. Differential diagnoses for compulsive hair pulling include OCD, Tourette's syndrome, and pervasive developmental disorders.

Semple DM *et al.*, eds. *Oxford Handbook of Psychiatry*, 1st edn. Oxford University Press, 2005, p. 387.

32. A.   There is a strong correlation between low IQ and incidence of schizophrenia. Traditionally, male and female incidences were thought to be equal but this has been recently challenged. McGrath undertook an exhaustive review of the literature on incidence rates and concluded that distribution of rates was significantly higher in males compared to females; the median male/female rate ratio was 1.40 in this analysis. Another meta-analysis, looking at 20 year's data on patients under 64, concluded similarly. Note that prevalence of schizophrenia does not differ between sexes. This may be because mortality is higher in males with schizophrenia.

Aleman A, Kahn RS, and Selten JP. Sex differences in the risk of schizophrenia: evidence from meta-analysis. *Archive of General Psychiatry* 2003; **60**: 565–571.

33. D. Though schizophrenia is equally prevalent in men and women, differences exist in the onset and course of illness. Onset and age at first hospitalization are earlier in men; women display a bimodal age distribution, with a second peak occurring in middle age. It is observed that men are more likely to be impaired by negative symptoms and women are more likely to have better premorbid adjustment. The outcome for female schizophrenia patients is better than that for male schizophrenia patients; currently it is unclear whether this could be attributed to later age of onset in females.

Sadock BJ and Sadock VA. *Kaplan & Sadock's Synopsis of Psychiatry: Behavioral Sciences/Clinical Psychiatry*, 10th edn. Lippincott Williams & Wilkins, 2007, p. 468.

34. B. The prevalence of schizophrenia in general population is around 1%. The prevalence rate increases when considering non-twin siblings of schizophrenia patients (8%). The risk is further elevated to 12% for a child born to a mother or father with schizophrenia. The risk shoots to 40% if both parents have schizophrenia, while having a monozygotic twin with schizophrenia increases the risk to 47% for the second twin. In dizygotic twins the risk is similar to that for a non-twin sibling, that is 12%.

Sadock BJ and Sadock VA. *Kaplan & Sadock's Synopsis of Psychiatry: Behavioral Sciences/Clinical Psychiatry*, 10th edn. Lippincott Williams & Wilkins, 2007, p. 471.

35. C. Velo–cardio–facial or di George syndrome (VCFS) is a genetic, autosomal dominant condition defined by Shprintzen in 1978. It occurs in 1 per 4000 live births; spontaneous deletion of chromosome 22q11.2 is responsible in most cases. It is characterised by mental retardation, facial dysmorphic features, cardiac anomalies, and neuroendocrine abnormalities, such as absent parathyroid, maldeveloped thymus, etc. It is thought to be related to problems in neural crest cell migration. Interestingly, the recent discovery of COMT polymorphism to be located at the same chromosomal loci adds to the speculation that psychosis is linked to this chromosome.

Chow EWC, Bassett AS, and Weksberg R. Velo-cardio-facial syndrome and psychotic disorders: implications for psychiatric genetics. *American Journal of Medical Genetics* 1994; **54**: 107–112.

36. B. The patient described in this question achieves sexual arousal by cross-dressing and retains heterosexual relationships. He is exhibiting fetishistic transvestism, a paraphilia or disorder of sexual preference. A patient with gender identity disorder will have dysphoria for biologically assigned gender (most often male sex) and will strongly prefer to change his appearance to that of opposite sex, through hormonal treatment or corrective surgeries. Sexual dysfunction of arousal phase refers to sexual aversion or lack of interest in having sexual intercourse. The scenario does not reflect the person's sexual orientation. Sexual orientation refers to homosexuality, heterosexuality, or bisexuality preference of an individual.

Gelder MG *et al.*, eds. *Shorter Oxford Textbook of Psychiatry*, 5th edn. Oxford University Press, 2006, p. 475.

37. C. The disorganised or hebephrenic schizophrenia is characterized by significant disruption in behaviour with some disinhibition. It characteristically has an earlier onset – around adolescence. These patients have pronounced formal thought disturbances, often with inappropriate emotional responses and incongruity of expression. In negative schizophrenia a deficit state starts without any positive psychotic symptoms. Residual schizophrenia is characterized by a history of florid positive symptoms in the past with current presentation suggestive of a negative syndrome. Schizoaffective disorder will have florid affective symptoms at the same time as prominent psychotic features.

Sadock BJ and Sadock VA. *Kaplan & Sadock's Synopsis of Psychiatry: Behavioral Sciences/Clinical Psychiatry*, 10th edn. Lippincott Williams & Wilkins, 2007, p. 477.

38. E. Cannabis intoxication can alter perceptual accuracy; colours may seem brighter with subjective slowing of the time. Depersonalization and derealization could occur. Cannabis-induced psychotic disorder is rare; transient paranoid ideation is more common. Hemp insanity refers to transient psychosis associated with heavy use of very potent cannabis. This is very rare and does not mimic schizophrenia in its course. It is generally believed that earlier onset of heavy potent cannabis use for a long duration can result in schizophrenia, at least in a group of genetically predisposed individuals. Cannabis can induce a sense of euphoria and relaxation, prompting self medication in patients with established schizophrenia.

Gelder MG *et al.*, eds. *New Oxford Textbook of Psychiatry*. Oxford University Press, 2000, p. 603.

39. C. Post schizophrenic depression is recognized in ICD-10 as a major depressive episode which starts within 12 months of the most recent psychotic episode; while residual psychotic symptoms can be present they must not be prominent. It is noted that such patients are likely to have had poor premorbid adjustment, schizoid traits, and more insidious onset of their psychotic symptoms. Family history of a mood disorder can increase the likelihood of developing post schizophrenic depression. It may be associated with a less-favourable prognosis, higher relapse, and a higher rate of suicide. DSM-IV TR considers postschizophrenic depression only as a research category.

World Health Organization. *The ICD-10 Classification of Mental and Behavioral Disorders; Clinical Descriptions and Diagnostic Guidelines*. Geneva: World Health Organization, 1992, p. 93

40. B. Persons with schizotypal (personality) disorder are strikingly peculiar, with magical thinking, occult beliefs, referential ideas, illusions, and obsessions without resistance. A significant number of patients claim paranormal experiences and clairvoyance. It occurs in about 3% of the population. A strikingly higher incidence is noted in those who are biological relatives of patients with schizophrenia. This disorder is so close to schizophrenia that ICD still includes schizotypal disorder together with other schizophrenia syndromes in Chapter F20–29.

Gelder MG *et al.*, eds. *New Oxford Textbook of Psychiatry*. Oxford University Press, 2000, p. 640.

41. B. In its natural course untreated depression lasts for 6 months while untreated mania lasts for about 4 months. So it is important that the therapy continues throughout this period as an absolute minimum. A manic episode by definition must meet a duration criteria of at least 1 week, or less if a patient must be hospitalized. A hypomanic episode must last at least 4 days. It is thought that as time goes, the intervals between episodes shorten, and the episodes themselves increase in duration. In a lifetime, patients with bipolar illness can have more than 10 episodes (both mania and depression) with duration and interepisodic interval stabilizing after the fourth or fifth episode.

Sadock BJ and Sadock VA. *Kaplan & Sadock's Synopsis of Psychiatry: Behavioral Sciences/Clinical Psychiatry*, 10th edn. Lippincott Williams & Wilkins, 2007, p. 550.

42. D. ICD-10 somatic syndrome includes: (1) loss of emotional reactivity; (2) diurnal mood variation; (3) anhedonia; (4) early morning awakening; (5) psychomotor agitation or retardation; (6) loss of appetite and weight; and (7) loss of libido. At least four symptoms must be definitely present to diagnose somatic syndrome.

World Health Organization. *The ICD-10 Classification of Mental and Behavioral Disorders; Clinical Descriptions and Diagnostic Guidelines*. Geneva: World Health Organization, 1992, p. 120.

43. A. The most appropriate diagnosis for this lady would be depressive disorder. According to the hierarchical organization of diagnoses, depression will trump a diagnosis of anxiety disorder. In this case, all of the mentioned features are well accounted for by depression itself. This lady fulfils two major criteria required for the diagnosis of depression. A diagnosis of mixed anxiety and depression is not coded in ICD-10.

World Health Organization. *The ICD-10 Classification of Mental and Behavioral Disorders; Clinical Descriptions and Diagnostic Guidelines.* Geneva: World Health Organization, 1992, p. 119.

44. B. Social phobia is characteristically more pronounced in smaller group setting where close scrutiny and criticism are more likely. The age of onset is around 15, much younger than other phobias. Blushing is seen as a part of anxiety symptoms in social phobia. In some cases a fear of losing control and vomiting in public is noted. Avoidance of group settings may lead to impaired social performance.

World Health Organization. *The ICD-10 Classification of Mental and Behavioral Disorders; Clinical Descriptions and Diagnostic Guidelines.* Geneva: World Health Organization, 1992, p. 137.

45. A. Hypercortisolaemia is seen in nearly 50% of those with major depression. This is evident by measuring excretion of urinary-free cortisol or salivary cortisol. It is posited that the normal feedback inhibition of ACTH and CRH by cortisol is disturbed due to abnormal glucocorticoid receptors, leading to high persistent cortisol levels. Dexamethasone administration (DST) fails to stimulate the feedback loop and so fails to suppress the cortisol level. This is one of the most consistent and robust findings in depression. But it is not specific to depression — it is also noted to some extent in mania, schizophrenia, dementia, and other psychiatric disorders.

Sadock BJ and Sadock VA. *Kaplan & Sadock's Synopsis of Psychiatry: Behavioral Sciences/Clinical Psychiatry*, 10th edn. Lippincott Williams & Wilkins, 2007, p. 531.

46. C. Life events are strong predictors of onset of depression. It is suggested that the association of life events and depression is stronger for the first episode than recurrences of depression. This may be because a kindling effect underlies depression. In other words, depression begets depression once the initial damage is done by a life event. It is not necessary that life events must precede the onset of depression in every patient.

Johnstone EC *et al.*, eds. *Companion to Psychiatric Studies*, 7th edn. Churchill Livingstone, 2004, p. 433.

47. C. In DSM-IV rapid cycling disorder is a course specifier while ICD-10 does not include this as a separate category or specifier. It can occur in both bipolar type I and bipolar type II disorders. Rapid cycling is diagnosed if there are at least four episodes fulfilling the criteria of major depression, mania, hypomania, or mixed mood disorder in the previous 12 months. Hypothyroidism is associated with rapid cycling bipolar disorder. Other causes of rapid cycling in a bipolar patient include the use of antidepressants that can induce switching, excessive use of stimulants including caffeine, non-compliance with medications, and presence of temporal lobe arrythmias in EEG. It is more common in women, in those with bipolar II, and can have a familial tendency to occur. Of bipolar patients, 5–15% can have rapid cycling at some point in their lifetime.

Kupka RW, Luckenbaugh DA, Post RM, *et al.* Rapid and non-rapid cycling bipolar disorder: A meta-analysis of clinical studies. *Journal of Clinical Psychiatry* 2003; **64**: 1483–1494.

48. E.   Good outcome in schizophrenia can be predicted by the presence of prominent affective symptoms during first presentation, acute onset, significant stressor at the onset, absence of family history of schizophrenia, good premorbid adjustment, having a family history of mood disorder, being female and living in a developing country.

Johnstone EC *et al.*, eds. *Companion to Psychiatric Studies*, 7th edn. Churchill Livingstone, 2004, p. 406; Box 19.6.

49. E.   In atypical depression mood is depressed but affect remains reactive. Vegetative signs may be characteristically reversed with hypersomnia, hyperphagia, reversed diurnal mood variation, leaden paralysis (a peculiar heaviness in the limbs), and hypersensitivity to rejection. Cognitive distortions of typical depression may be absent. The characterization of this subgroup of depression is owed largely to an observation that the effects of MAO inhibitors such as phenelzine are better than other antidepressants in this population.

Semple DM *et al.*, eds. *Oxford Handbook of Psychiatry*, 1st edn. Oxford University Press, 2005, p. 268.

50. C.   Heritability of bipolar disorder was estimated as 85% by McGuffin *et al.* Variable rates are reported in other studies. Currently, it is generally accepted that bipolar disorder is one of the most heritable psychiatric disorders.

McGuffin P, Rijsdijk F, Andrew M, *et al.* The heritability of bipolar affective disorder and the genetic relationship to unipolar depression. *Archives of General Psychiatry* 2003; **60**: 497–502.

51. B.   Bipolar disorder starts with depression in up to 70% of patients. In a small proportion (10–20%) only recurrent mania is observed (still classed as bipolar under DSM); 90% of those who experienced mania are likely to have another, while the remaining 10% have only one episode of mania throughout their lifetime.

Sadock BJ and Sadock VA. *Kaplan & Sadock's Synopsis of Psychiatry: Behavioral Sciences/Clinical Psychiatry*, 10th edn. Lippincott Williams & Wilkins, 2007, p. 550.

52. A.   The concept tested here is that any patient who has psychotic features in a background of elated mood has mania irrespective of the duration criteria. Also remember that any patient with elation and psychosocial impairment that necessitates hospitalization is diagnosed to have mania and not hypomania according to DSM-IV, irrespective of the duration criteria. In the absence of psychotic symptoms or hospitalization, clinical features must last for at least 7 days before a manic episode can be diagnosed.

Johnstone EC *et al.*, eds. *Companion to Psychiatric Studies*, 7th edn. Churchill Livingstone, 2004, p. 427.

53. A.   Delusions of all types can present in bipolar disorder, as they do in schizophrenia. Family history of affective disorders is not uncommon in patients with schizophrenia, invalidating this aspect as a strong feature to differentiate the two major psychoses. Cannabis use and religious hallucinations can also occur in bipolar disorder. Ever since Kraeplinian concept of dementia praecox was introduced, one reasonable, though not always reliable, feature that differentiates these two illnesses is the absence of interepisodic residual symptoms in bipolar disorder. In the majority of patients with schizophrenia significant impairment is noted even between full-blown psychotic episodes. But note that residual cognitive impairment is increasingly noted in euthymic bipolar patients.

Gelder MG *et al.*, eds. *New Oxford Textbook of Psychiatry*. Oxford University Press, 2000, p. 568.

54.A. Bipolar disorder has no gender variation in prevalence rates. Unipolar depressive disorder is more common in women of all ages compared to men. The only time in life where the incidence is equal or slightly higher in males is when depression is prepubertal, and this is rare. The gender gap narrows with advancing age and in geriatric population the incidence rates across the genders are very much closer than in early adult life. Rapid cycling is more common in women, for unknown reasons.

Johnstone EC et al., eds. Companion to Psychiatric Studies, 7th edn. Churchill Livingstone, 2004, p. 429.

55.B. Bipolar is the most heritable of all psychiatric disorders. Apart from being a risk factor for the development of bipolar disorder, a family history of bipolar disorder increases the risk for any mood disorders. Overall, in families of patients with bipolar illness, unipolar depression is the most common expressed phenotype. Note that a significant proportion of these unipolar patients can later get a revised diagnosis of bipolar disorder. Thus the mood disorders do not breed true on their own. The heritability of schizophrenia is around 50–60%. Conduct disorders and alcoholism have lower heritability rates than the psychoses.

Sadock BJ and Sadock VA. Kaplan & Sadock's Synopsis of Psychiatry: Behavioral Sciences/Clinical Psychiatry, 10th edn. Lippincott Williams & Wilkins, 2007, p. 532.

56.C. Double depression refers to an episode of major depression in a patient with dysthymia. Dysthymic disorder is distinguished from major depressive disorder using both severity and duration criteria. Dysthymic patients complain that they have always been depressed since childhood or adolescence. A patient with dysthymia is prone to get recurrent depression, and major depression of various severities can occur on top of dysthymia, leading to double depression. It is estimated that nearly 40% of patients with major depression actually have a double depression. The prognosis may be poor in double depression.

Sadock BJ and Sadock VA. Kaplan & Sadock's Synopsis of Psychiatry: Behavioral Sciences/Clinical Psychiatry, 10th edn. Lippincott Williams & Wilkins, 2007, p. 565.

57.A. Antineuronal antibodies are produced by group A beta haemolytic streptococci infection. This damages caudate nucleus resulting in Sydenham's chorea. Also, patients with Sydenham's chorea often have obsessive and compulsive symptoms, emotional lability, and hyperactivity. This is a spectrum of paediatric autoimmune neuropsychiatric disorders associated with streptococcal infections (PANDAS). Guillain–Barré syndrome is an acute demyelinating disease of peripheral nerves.

Gelder MG et al., eds. New Oxford Textbook of Psychiatry. Oxford University Press, 2000, p. 825.

58.D. Among various risk factors attributed to the aetiology of depression, family history, neuroticism, recent life stressor, and past history of depression have most evidence. Brown and Harris in a landmark study established high risk of depression in urban-living women with early maternal loss, lack of a confiding relationship, greater than three children under the age of 14 at home, and unemployment.

Patten SB. Are the Brown and Harris vulnerability factors risk factors for depression? Journal of Psychiatry and Neuroscience 1991; **16**: 267–271.
Gelder MG et al., eds. New Oxford Textbook of Psychiatry. Oxford University Press, 2000, p. 698.

59.C. Patients with obsessions usually harbour their difficulties for a long time (often 5 to 10 years) before they present to a doctor. The ego-dystonic nature of obsessions results in anxiety and reduces help seeking and sharing of their secret illness. OCD has its origin in adolescence or childhood. But most patients do not seek help until they are in their twenties or thirties. Often the onset of depression brings OCD to clinical attention.

Gelder MG et al., eds. New Oxford Textbook of Psychiatry. Oxford University Press, 2000, p. 824.

60. A. Probable pointers in this vignette suggesting a diagnosis of schizophrenia are: (1) age of onset and (2) ideas of ego alien thought insertion. Prodrome of psychosis may present with obsessional symptoms. Often it is difficult to differentiate OCD from schizophrenia in such presentations. But the useful pointers are: (1) ego-dystonic nature of obsessions may not be prominent in psychosis; (2) insight that the thoughts are one's own may not be seen in psychosis; (3) resistance to the obsessions may be conspicuously absent; and (4) content of obsessions may be bizarre, instead of the usual themes of safety, contamination, sex, violence, religion, etc.

Gelder MG *et al.*, eds. *New Oxford Textbook of Psychiatry*. Oxford University Press, 2000, p. 824.

61. B. Night terror is a sleep disorder seen mostly in children. It is a disturbance of slow wave non-REM sleep. Generally in NREM sleep, dreams cannot be fully recollected. When a patient wakes up from NREM sleep, he is often confused. A night terror is a dramatic episode where the patient screams, has autonomic arousal, appears confused but goes back to sleep without clear memory of the arousal the next morning. Though this is fairly common in children around age 7, a new onset sleep terror in adults should prompt neurological investigations to rule out epilepsy or brain damage. About 1 to 6% of children have the disorder. It is more common in boys and tends to run in families.

Johnstone EC *et al.*, eds. *Companion to Psychiatric Studies*, 7th edn. Churchill Livingstone, 2004, p. 785.

62. C. Irrational fears are common in childhood but most of them disappear by adolescence. Any irrational fear of certain objects or situations associated with strong avoidance behaviour prompts a diagnosis of phobia. Phobia can develop against any object/ place though certain phobias, for example animals or spider phobia, seem common and more recurring than others; this might have an evolutionary explanation (stimulus preparedness).

World Health Organization. *The ICD-10 Classification of Mental and Behavioral Disorders; Clinical Descriptions and Diagnostic Guidelines*. Geneva: World Health Organization, 1992, p. 138.

63. C. Blood injury injection phobia is different from other phobias in two important aspects: (1) the autonomic response to exposure is low blood pressure, bradycardia, and fainting response instead of the more common tachycardia, increased blood pressure, and flight response; and (2) there is a strong genetic component in the aetiology of blood injury injection type of phobia. The affected persons may have inherited a particularly strong vasovagal reflex, which becomes associated with phobic emotions.

Sadock BJ and Sadock VA. *Kaplan & Sadock's Synopsis of Psychiatry: Behavioral Sciences/Clinical Psychiatry*, 10th edn. Lippincott Williams & Wilkins, 2007, p. 600.

64. B. Emotional numbing when undergoing the trauma is associated with later risk of developing PTSD. PTSD occurs after exposure to stressful event of exceptionally threatening or catastrophic nature. But not everyone who is exposed to such situations develops PTSD. Predisposing factors may include pre-existing neuroticism, genetic predisposition (one-third of the variance is explained by genes), and hypocortisolaemia apart from an abnormal hippocampal response to stress.

Feeny NC *et al.* Exploring the roles of emotional numbing, depression, and dissociation in PTSD. *Journal of Traumatic Stress* 2000; **13**: 489–498.

65. E. Panic attacks have an autonomic arousal component with sweating, palpitation, trembling or shaking, shortness of breath or smothering, feeling of choking, nausea, and dizziness. A cognitive component is characterized by fear of going mad, losing control, fear of dying, derealization and depersonalization. The most characteristic type of panic attack is the spontaneous (out of the blue) episode. Situational panic attacks occur when exposed to or anticipating an exposure to a particular situations. Occasionally, some individuals have panic attacks in certain situations sometimes but not always – these are called situationally predisposed panic attacks. Nocturnal panic attacks are common in patients with panic disorder. They are similar to panic attacks that occur in daytime. Isolated, nocturnal panic attacks are rare and must prompt investigations to rule out medical causes. Especially in case of non-fearful panic attacks where cognitive components are absent, one should suspect medical causes. There is nothing called unilateral panic attack!

Gelder MG et al., eds. New Oxford Textbook of Psychiatry. Oxford University Press, 2000, p. 807.

66. C. Behavioural inhibition to the unfamiliar is a temperamental construct that refers to a characteristic propensity to react to both social and non-social novelty with inhibition. In contrast, shyness refers to feelings of discomfort in social situations but not non-social situations. Extreme behavioural inhibition is also denoted as neophobia. Some children have a consistent pattern of behavioural inhibition, especially if parents have an anxiety disorder themselves. This may grow into social phobia in at least some.

Van Ameringen M et al. The relationship of behavioral inhibition and shyness to anxiety disorder. Journal of Nervous and Mental Disease 1998; **186**: 425–431.

67. A. Panic disorder has higher prevalence in females than males at a ratio of 3:2 in community samples and 3:1 in clinical samples. The onset of panic disorder falls into two peaks – the first occurs in the early to mid-twenties (15–24 years) with a second peak at around 50 (45–54 years). The onset of panic disorder for the first time in elderly people is extremely rare.

Gelder MG et al., eds. New Oxford Textbook of Psychiatry. Oxford University Press, 2000, p. 811.

68. D. The phenomenology of grief is very similar to depression, but some important differentiating features exist. For example though all features of somatic syndrome, guilt regarding the death, and preoccupation with the unfortunate event occurs in normal grief, recurrent suicidal ideas, psychomotor retardation, inappropriate guilt not pertaining to the loss, and psychotic symptoms other than transient visual hallucination of the loved one are unusual. These symptoms, if present, warrant a diagnosis of abnormal grief/ major depressive episode.

Gelder MG et al., eds. New Oxford Textbook of Psychiatry. Oxford University Press, 2000, p. 1144.

69. E. Brown and Harris, in a landmark study, established the high risk of depression in urban-living women with early maternal loss, lack of a confiding relationship, greater than three children under the age of 14 at home, and unemployment. Though urban living is not quoted as one of the four identified factors, it is important to note that the study was carried out in Camberwell, an inner city area with high deprivation rates.

Patten SB. Are the Brown and Harris vulnerability factors risk factors for depression? Journal of Psychiatry and Neuroscience 1991; **16**: 267–271.

70. A. According to ICD-10 criteria for PTSD to be diagnosed the cluster of hyperarousal, flashbacks, irritability and intrusive memories must occur within 6 months of the traumatic event. A diagnosis of probable PTSD can be made after 6 month's interval. This is largely an arbitrary cut off without much difference in clinical features of the two groups.

World Health Organization. The ICD-10 Classification of Mental and Behavioral Disorders; Clinical Descriptions and Diagnostic Guidelines. Geneva: World Health Organization, 1992, p. 148.

71. D. It is observed that about 20–30% of those with OCD show a significant improvement, 40–50% have a moderate improvement, while the rest have a chronic or worsening course. Poor prognostic factors include yielding to compulsions, a childhood onset, bizarre content of compulsions, need for hospitalization, a coexisting major depressive disorder, the presence of overvalued ideas, and the presence of personality disorder (especially schizotypal). A good prognosis is indicated by good premorbid adjustment, the presence of a precipitating event, and episodic nature. The content or theme of obsessions and family history do not relate to the prognosis.

Gelder MG et al., eds. *New Oxford Textbook of Psychiatry*. Oxford University Press, 2000, p. 824.

72. A. The most common method of self harm attempt in the UK is paracetamol overdose. In the UK, self poisoning by drugs accounts for nearly 90% all hospital presentations with self harm. The next most common method of self harm is cutting wrists. The most common method employed in those successfully committing suicide is hanging. In general, violent methods such as hanging or use of firearms are common among male victims of suicide. Self immolation is associated with schizophrenia, south Asian women, and combined suicide–homicides. Presence of mental illness increases the severity of suicide attempt. Tricyclic antidepressant-related death was more common in the past but has reduced following a reduction in prescriptions.

Johnstone EC et al., eds. *Companion to Psychiatric Studies*, 7th edn. Churchill Livingstone, 2004, p. 671.

73. C. Sixty-six percent of suicide victims are seen by their general practitioner in the month prior to suicide. Nearly 40% have seen their GP in the week preceding death. One-quarter of suicide victims are on an active psychiatric out-patient list at the time of death. Half of these have seen their psychiatrists in the week preceding death.

Appleby L, Shaw J, Amos T, et al. *Safer Services. Report of the National Confidential Inquiry into Suicide and Homicide by People with Mental Illness*. London: Department of Health, 1999.

74. D. Features of paranoid personality disorder include pervasive distrust and suspiciousness, reading hidden self-referential meaning from benign events, bearing grudges persistently, and a tenacious sense of personal rights and suspicion of infringement on those rights leading to quarrelsome and litigious tendency.

World Health Organization. *The ICD-10 Classification of Mental and Behavioral Disorders; Clinical Descriptions and Diagnostic Guidelines*. Geneva: World Health Organization, 1992, p. 203.

75. C. Patients with schizoid personality display a pervasive pattern of detachment from social relationships and a restricted range of emotional expression. They do not desire close relationships and prefer to be solitary with almost absent sexual interest. They lack close confidants and appear indifferent to both praise and criticism by others. Inability to plan ahead is seen in antisocial personality, while borderline and avoidant personalities show sensitivity to rejection. Narcissistic individuals may have a sense of excessive self importance. Impulsivity and lack of self restraint are seen in both antisocial and borderline personality disorders.

Gelder MG et al., eds. *New Oxford Textbook of Psychiatry*. Oxford University Press, 2000, p. 929.

76. A   Histrionic personality disorder is characterized by a high degree of attention-seeking behaviour, craving for attention, and sexualizing and seductive behaviour even in professional or non-social settings. These patients tend to have rather superficial relationships. They tend to display rapidly shifting and shallow expression of emotions. In addition, they have a style of speech that is excessively impressionistic and lacking in detail with self-dramatization and artificially exaggerated emotional expression. They may be highly suggestible too. People with narcissistic personality are not particularly attention seeking in their behaviour. But similar to those with histrionic traits, individuals with narcissistic traits have shallow expression of emotions. In addition, they have a strong need for admiration together with a sense of self importance. Body image disturbances are seen in those with borderline personality traits, along with disturbed self identity. But excessive concern with physical appearance is not characteristic of borderline personality.

Sadock BJ and Sadock VA. *Kaplan & Sadock's Synopsis of Psychiatry: Behavioral Sciences/Clinical Psychiatry*, 10th edn. Lippincott Williams & Wilkins, 2007, p. 802.

77. A.   The characteristic behaviour of the avoidant personality is active isolation from the social environment. But in contrast to schizoid personality, where passive social isolation is seen, avoidant patients isolate to protect themselves because they are extremely sensitive to rejection.

Gelder MG *et al.*, eds. *New Oxford Textbook of Psychiatry*. Oxford University Press, 2000, p. 942.

78. A.   Borderline personality disorder is characterized by affective instability, impulsivity, chronic emptiness, sensitivity to rejection resulting in intense relationships that are often short lived, and micropsychotic episodes induced by stressful events. It is increasingly speculated that borderline disorder exists in a spectrum which at its most severe pole includes bipolar illness. Various observations provide preliminary support to this claim. Family history of bipolar illness is more common in borderline personality disorder; development of bipolar illness on follow up is higher in borderline than any other personality disorders; affective instability and impulsivity are important features of both borderline disorder and bipolar illness.

Magill CA. The boundary between borderline personality disorder and bipolar disorder: current concepts and challenges. *Canadian Journal of Psychiatry* 2004; **49**: 551–556.

79. C.   The relationship between obsessive–compulsive personality disorder and obsessive–compulsive disorder is controversial. Though it was suggested that most obsessive–compulsive personality disorder become obsessive–compulsive disorder in later life, recent studies refute this. Among various psychiatric disorders that may present in a patient with obsessive personality, depressive and anxiety disorders are the most common, followed by phobic, somatoform, and obsessive–compulsive symptoms.

Gelder MG *et al.*, eds. *New Oxford Textbook of Psychiatry*. Oxford University Press, 2000, p. 945.

80. B. Most patients with schizophrenia who commit suicide are in an acute phase of psychosis, have a history of previous attempt, achieve poor symptom control, have a high degree of comorbidity, and show greater non-compliance. For several decades, the literature has quoted the lifetime risk of suicide in schizophrenia as 10–15% (from Miles *et al.* who examined mortality reports published between 1931 and 1975, and estimated the lifetime risk to be 10%). This figure was subsequently challenged by Inskip *et al.* who analysed 29 studies using proportionate mortality (the percentage of the dead who died by suicide) and estimated the risk to be substantially lower at 4%. A recent meta-analysis by Palmer *et al.*, using more rigorous methods, has concluded that the rate of suicide in schizophrenia is around 5.6%.

Palmer BA, Pankratz VS, and Bostwick JM. The lifetime risk of suicide in schizophrenia: a reexamination. *Archives of General Psychiatry* 2005; **62**: 247–253.

Miles CP. Conditions predisposing to suicide: a review. *Journal of Nervous and Mental Disease* 1977; **164**: 231–246.

Inskip HM, Harris EC, Barraclough B. Lifetime risk of suicide for affective disorder, alcoholism and schizophrenia. *British Journal of Psychiatry* 1998; **172**: 35–37.

81. A. It was widely believed that schizophrenia is a universal illness with a more or less equivalent global prevalence of 1%. McGrath and colleagues have recently challenged this figure. Compiling data from nearly 200 studies that reported on epidemiology of schizophrenia, they estimated the mean lifetime prevalence of schizophrenia (the proportion of individuals in the population who have ever manifested the illness and who are alive on a given day) as 4 per 1000. Note that DSM-IV states that the lifetime prevalence of schizophrenia is often reported to be 5 to15 per 1000. McGrath and colleagues also determined that the point prevalence of schizophrenia (the proportion of individuals who manifest the illness at a given point of time) is 4.6 per 1000. The lifetime morbid risk of schizophrenia (the probability of a person developing the illness during his or her lifetime) is determined to be at a rate of 7 per 1000 (nearly 1 in 150 as mentioned in the question).

Saha S, Chant D, Welham J, and McGrath J. A systematic review of the prevalence of schizophrenia. *PLoS Medicine*; **2**: e141 doi:10.1371/journal.pmed.0020141.

82. B. Narcolepsy is characterized by irresistible attacks of sleep together with cataplexy (brief episodes of sudden bilateral loss of muscle tone, often in association with intense emotion) and recurrent hypnapompic or hypnagogic hallucinations or sleep paralysis at the beginning or end of a sleep episode. Characteristically, the EEG shows REM pattern during hypnagogic or hypnapompic hallucinations and sleep paralysis. The narcoleptic sleep is usually a refreshing (REM) sleep. Sleep onset REM is characteristic. Strong genetic association with HLA-DR2 locus is noted, with an autosomal dominant inheritance. HLA-DR2 is found in 90 to 100% of patients with narcolepsy. It is also shown that patients with narcolepsy are deficient in the neurotransmitter hypocretin (also called orexin) associated with hypothalamic modulation of appetite and alertness. EEG is normal between narcoleptic attacks.

Sadock BJ and Sadock VA. *Kaplan & Sadock's Synopsis of Psychiatry: Behavioral Sciences/Clinical Psychiatry*, 10th edn. Lippincott Williams & Wilkins, 2007, p. 760.

83. B. Sleepwalking or somnambulism consists of various complex motor behaviours during the first third of sleep where slow wave NREM (stage III and IV) phase predominates. Usually, the patient will not retain any memory of getting up and walking during sleep. The motor acts are often perseverative in nature; incidence is most common around age 12.

Sadock BJ and Sadock VA. *Kaplan & Sadock's Synopsis of Psychiatry: Behavioral Sciences/Clinical Psychiatry*, 10th edn. Lippincott Williams & Wilkins, 2007, p. 767.

84. C. Both mania and depression are characterized by various neurovegetative signs – disturbances in sleep, appetite, weight, energy levels, and circadian functions. In depression early morning awakening is characteristic. To qualify as early morning awakening, a patient must wake up at least 2 hours prior to his usual waking time. In mania, there is increased energy associated with reduced need for sleep. Patients can go on for many days with barely any sleep. Paradoxically, sleep deprivation itself can induce a state similar to hypomania in some susceptible individuals.

World Health Organization. *The ICD-10 Classification of Mental and Behavioral Disorders; Clinical Descriptions and Diagnostic Guidelines.* Geneva: World Health Organization, 1992, p. 114.

85. D. Panic attacks can occur in various medical conditions such as hyperthyroidism, phaeochromocytoma, epilepsy, cardiac arrhythmias, and chronic obstructive pulmonary disease. It is also noted that some medical conditions occur slightly more commonly in those with panic disorder, for example mitral valve prolapse, hyperthyroidism.

Gelder MG *et al.*, eds. *New Oxford Textbook of Psychiatry.* Oxford University Press, 2000, p. 810.

86. A. Bulimia nervosa and anorexia nervosa are not mutually exclusive disorders. Significant overlap occurs between the two and also with EDNOS (eating disorder not otherwise specified). In bulimia, more impulsivity and less perfectionist traits are noted. Bulimia nervosa is characterized by higher rates of partial and full recovery compared with anorexia nervosa. Both anorexia and bulimia cannot be diagnosed at the same time as a range of bulimic behaviours are described under the diagnosis of anorexia itself.

Johnstone EC *et al.*, eds. *Companion to Psychiatric Studies*, 7th edn. Churchill Livingstone, 2004, p. 498.

87. A. In some elderly patients with depression, marked difficulties with concentration and memory can present similar to dementia. Presence of previous history of depression; clearly observable depressed mood; biological symptoms of depression; voluntary complaints about memory failure (patients with dementia tend not to realize their own memory problems); indifference and 'I don't know' answers when formally testing memory (while confabulation may be seen in dementia); and response to antidepressant medication (unusual in true dementia) are some clues to pseudodementia. In cognitive tests, visuospatial and executive functions can be impaired in dementia but such impairment is highly unlikely to be due to isolated depression. Neurological signs, including frontal release, points towards dementia.

Sadock BJ and Sadock VA. *Kaplan & Sadock's Synopsis of Psychiatry: Behavioral Sciences/Clinical Psychiatry*, 10th edn. Lippincott Williams & Wilkins, 2007, p. 339; Table 10.3–11.

88. D. Paraphrenia is a late-onset psychotic disorder characterized by persecutory and referential delusions with or without auditory hallucinations. It is believed to be a very-late-onset (>60) variant of schizophrenia as many patients with a family history of schizophrenia show an increased rate of paraphrenia. Negative symptoms are conspicuously absent in paraphrenia. Schneiderian first-rank symptoms are uncommon too.

Gelder MG *et al.*, eds. *New Oxford Textbook of Psychiatry.* Oxford University Press, 2000, p. 1642.

89. D. According to DSM-IV-TR, dissociative identity disorder (multiple personality disorder) is characterized by the presence of two or more distinct identities or personality states that recurrently take control of the individual's behaviour. The patient cannot recall important personal information that occurs when the alternate personality is in control (one-way amnesia). The personality states are also called alters. Often alters are widely different in their perception, relation, and adaptation to the environment and self. This controversial and dramatic condition is placed under dissociative disorders in both ICD and DSM.

World Health Organization. *The ICD-10 Classification of Mental and Behavioral Disorders; Clinical Descriptions and Diagnostic Guidelines.* Geneva: World Health Organization, 1992, p. 160.

90. D.   Dissociative fugue is characterized by sudden, unexpected but purposeful travel away from one's routine dwelling, associated with amnesia for strikingly significant periods of the past. This may be associated with assumption of a new identity. Though this can occur in depression, it is more often seen as stress-induced dissociation state. Depersonalization is not a characteristic accompaniment. Family history of epilepsy in a patient with fugue state must prompt investigations for TLE. Usually, patients with fugue have no anterograde amnesia or attention difficulties and have apparently good self care and social interaction.

World Health Organization. *The ICD-10 Classification of Mental and Behavioral Disorders; Clinical Descriptions and Diagnostic Guidelines*. Geneva: World Health Organization, 1992, p. 155.

91. E.   In chronic fatigue syndrome (also called myalgic encephalomyelitis or postviral fatigue; described as neurasthenia in ICD-10) the central feature is severe fatigue which is not related to level of exertion and unrelieved by rest. This is accompanied by aching muscles, insomnia, aching joints, and irritability. Patient may complain of sore throat, fever, and tender lymph nodes, especially, retrospectively, around the time of onset.

Gelder MG *et al.*, eds. *New Oxford Textbook of Psychiatry*. Oxford University Press, 2000, p. 1113.

92. D.   There are important conceptual differences between somatization disorder and hypochondriasis. In hypochondriasis the patient dreads the presence of an undiagnosed disorder. He seeks diagnosis more than treatment. The patient asks for various unwarranted diagnostic tests but will not be satisfied by any negative results. A patient with somatization is not concerned about diagnosis as much as she is concerned about symptom relief and intervention. Various sophisticated diagnostic measures are not sought usually. Instead, various treatments may be tried by both patients and health-care professionals.

World Health Organization. *The ICD-10 Classification of Mental and Behavioral Disorders; Clinical Descriptions and Diagnostic Guidelines*. Geneva: World Health Organization, 1992, pp. 162, 164.

93. E.   Multiple sclerosis can present with discrete neurological dysfunctions separated in both time and bodily location. These symptoms often resolve on their own (relapsing–remitting course). For example, as in this case, bladder dysfunction and limb weakness. Conversion disorder also presents with neurological dysfunction (often 'loss of function' as opposed to somatoform disorder where there is a 'positive' symptom such as pain) which can resolve on its own, on resolution of a conflict.

World Health Organization. *The ICD-10 Classification of Mental and Behavioral Disorders; Clinical Descriptions and Diagnostic Guidelines*. Geneva: World Health Organization, 1992, p. 158.

94. C.   Past history of suicidal attempt is the most important predictor of risk. Other risk factors include family history of suicide, history of a major mental illness, low socioeconomic status, postdischarge period, severe physical illness, and easy access to lethal methods.

Gelder MG *et al.*, eds. *New Oxford Textbook of Psychiatry*. Oxford University Press, 2000, p. 1035.

95. B.   This is a difficult question; questions of this type are best answered at their face value, with only the given information and without making any further assumptions . Patient A has obsessional symptoms with no other pathology highlighted. As such, the risk of suicide is low in OCD without depression. Patient C has the risk factor of alcohol use, but the rest of the history (female, young, sought help, impulsive) suggests low risk. Patients D and E seem to have no suicidal intention. Patient B has various risk factors – middle aged, male, had a violent attempt, and a widower.

Gelder MG *et al.*, eds. *New Oxford Textbook of Psychiatry*. Oxford University Press, 2000, p. 1035.

96. A.   A major depressive episode is found in approximately 10% of patients, while nearly 50 to 75% show some features of subclinical depression. Depression reported by carers can range up to 85%. Depression is more common in the early than in the later stages of AD – this may be due to preserved insight during early stages or because of the fact that clinical assessment of depression becomes more difficult when dementia worsens.

Gelder MG *et al.*, eds. *New Oxford Textbook of Psychiatry*. Oxford University Press, 2000, p. 389.

97. A.   Malingering is often not considered seriously in general clinical practice. Though it may be difficult to establish, it should be suspected whenever obvious discrepancies exist in historical accounts and observed signs. Amnesia for the content of hallucinatory voices is distinctly unusual.

Gelder MG *et al.*, eds. *New Oxford Textbook of Psychiatry*. Oxford University Press, 2000, p. 1129.

98. B.   Kleine–Levin syndrome is characterized by recurrent episodes of prolonged sleep intermingled with periods of normal sleep. During the prolonged sleep phases, social withdrawal, apathy, irritability, and megaphagia (increased eating) can occur. Unexplained fever may occur in such patients. This is a rare illness with onset between the ages of 10 and 21 years. It is mostly self-limiting. Curiously, this is a favourite theme tested in MRCPsych exams!

Sadock BJ and Sadock VA. *Kaplan & Sadock's Synopsis of Psychiatry: Behavioral Sciences/Clinical Psychiatry*, 10th edn. Lippincott Williams & Wilkins, 2007, p. 765.

99. D.   REM behavioural disorder refers to episodes of complex, sometimes violent acting out of dreams. It is common in older men with a history of brain ischaemia. It can appear as an early event in the evolution of Parkinson's disease or Lewy body dementia. Polysomnography shows failure of normal REM related hypotonia.

Sadock BJ and Sadock VA. *Kaplan & Sadock's Synopsis of Psychiatry: Behavioral Sciences/Clinical Psychiatry*, 10th edn. Lippincott Williams & Wilkins, 2007, p. 768.

100. C.   Absence seizures can mimic thought blocking. Absence seizure is a type of generalized seizure where the episodes may often go unnoticed due to a lack of dramatic motor or sensory symptoms. Also called petit mal epilepsy, it usually begins in childhood and stops by puberty. A patient with absence seizures has a very brief loss of consciousness which can occur numerous times in a single day (up to 100 in some cases). EEG produces a characteristic pattern of three-per-second spike-and-wave.

Sadock BJ and Sadock VA. *Kaplan & Sadock's Synopsis of Psychiatry: Behavioral Sciences/Clinical Psychiatry*, 10th edn. Lippincott Williams & Wilkins, 2007, p. 360.

1. **Description and categorization of abnormal experiences as reported by the patient and observed from his behaviour is known as**
   A. Experimental psychopathology
   B. Descriptive psychopathology
   C. Explanatory psychopathology
   D. Philosophical psychiatry
   E. None of the above

2. **A 55-year-old man with chronic schizophrenia resists any passive limb movements attempted during a neurological examination, in spite of being asked not to do so. Which of the following symptom is he exhibiting?**
   A. Obstruction
   B. Negativism
   C. Automatic obedience
   D. Waxy flexibility
   E. Ambitendency

3. **According to Jaspers, the most important component of psychiatric assessment is**
   A. Empathy
   B. Humour
   C. Judgement
   D. Reasoning
   E. Common sense

4. **The concept of symptoms assessed by descriptive psychopathology has both form and content as its components. Which of the following, with regard to this statement, is true?**
   A. Form provides sufficient information for management
   B. Form provides sufficient information for severity
   C. Form is more important than content
   D. Form provides sufficient information for diagnosis
   E. Content is more important than form

5. **A patient is experiencing increased brightness and acuity of visual objects. Intense perceptions occur in all of the following EXCEPT**

    A. Migraine
    B. Hallucinogens
    C. Mania
    D. Delirium
    E. Depression

6. **A 35-year-old lady complains of changes in the shape of objects perceived. She is having difficulties in perceiving the symmetry of objects. This symptom is called**

    A. Dysmegalopsia
    B. Micropsia
    C. Macropsia
    D. Lilliputian hallucinations
    E. Pareidolia

7. **A 12-year-old boy, at a school anniversary celebration, vividly describes what martians may look like. Which of the following is true about this imagery? The imagery is**

    A. A perception
    B. A fantasy
    C. A pseudohallucination
    D. An illusion
    E. None of the above

8. **An 8-year-old boy is frightened to be alone at home. He starts seeing monsters out of wind moving through window curtains. Which of the following symptoms is he experiencing?**

    A. Pareidolia
    B. Completion illusion
    C. Eidetic imagery
    D. Affect illusion
    E. Hallucination

9. **A 19-year-old man sees his new girlfriend's face from the shapes of clouds. This perception will**

    A. Intensify on paying attention
    B. Cannot be dismissed voluntarily
    C. Arises from unambiguous stimuli
    D. Associated with intense affect change
    E. Associated with loss of insight

10. **A 35-year-old lady reports hearing voices in her head. Which of the following differences between hallucination and pseudohallucination is true?**

A. In true hallucinations insight is often retained
B. True hallucinations are often identified to be originating from self
C. True hallucinations occur in subjective space
D. True hallucinations are sought in other modalities by the patient
E. True hallucinations cannot occur in two modalities simultaneously

11. **Which one of the following is an elementary hallucination?**

A. Flashes of light
B. Visions of small mice in a minutiae
C. Voices repeating the word 'go'
D. Voices speaking in an unknown language
E. None of the above

12. **Which of the following is NOT a common feature of schizophrenic auditory hallucinations?**

A. Being multiple
B. Male voice
C. Speaks in one's mother tongue
D. Often continuously present
E. Has a different accent

13. **Which of the following can cause visual hallucinations?**

A. Occipital lobe tumours
B. Postconcussion states
C. Hepatic failure
D. Dementia
E. All of the above

14. **An 80-year-old lady with normal consciousness experiences vivid, distinct, colourful images of Mickey Mouse in her living room. On physical examination one must look for which of the following signs?**

A. Visual acuity
B. Glasgow coma scale
C. Plantar reflex
D. Knee jerk
E. Cranial nerves

15. **A patient withdrawing from alcohol sees small Chinese soldiers marching on his carpet. This phenomenon is called**

A. Micropsia
B. Macropsia
C. Lilliputian hallucination
D. Pseudohallucination
E. Affective illusion

16. **A 22-year-old college student reports a peculiar visual disturbance that causes images to persist even after their corresponding stimulus has ceased. Which of the following symptoms best suits the above description?**

    A. Pareidolia
    B. Palinopsia
    C. Autoscopy
    D. Imagery
    E. Formication

17. **A 54-year-old man who is living at a psychiatric rehabilitation home complains of seeing his own image outside his body. Which of the following is the commonest psychiatric cause of this phenomenon?**

    A. Schizophrenia
    B. Temporal lobe epilepsy
    C. Depression
    D. Mania
    E. Dementia

18. **Which of the following drugs on withdrawal produce disturbed proprioceptive perceptions?**

    A. Cannabis
    B. Amphetamines
    C. LSD
    D. Benzodiazepines
    E. Nicotine

19. **A patient, whose right arm was amputated following a crush injury, suffers from recurrent, tactile sensations arising out of the lost limb. Which of the following symptoms is this description classified as?**

    A. Hallucination
    B. Pseudohallucination
    C. Body image disturbance
    D. Somatization
    E. Delusion

20. **Which of the following is an extracampine hallucination?**

    A. A 45-year-old man hears voices coming from the South Pole
    B. A 33-year-old man hears a voice coming from his left knee
    C. A 56-year-old lady sees a devil's tail hanging on a hook
    D. A 31-year-old man sees an angel without a face
    E. None of the above

21. **A patient can hear voices when ever the noise of water running through a tap is heard. This is called**
    A. Reflex hallucination
    B. Synaesthesia
    C. Functional hallucination
    D. Extracampine hallucination
    E. Reverse hallucination

22. **The phenomenon of perceiving a stimulus of one modality in a different modality is called**
    A. Reflex hallucination
    B. Synaesthesia
    C. Functional hallucination
    D. Extracampine hallucination
    E. Reverse hallucination

23. **An 18-year-old girl is able to perceive colours when she listens to cello music. Which of the following is incorrect regarding synaesthesia?**
    A. It is more common in females
    B. It is often occurs in multiple members of a family
    C. Colour–number synaesthesia is the most common type.
    D. It is related to defective synaptic pruning
    E. It is a form of hallucination

24. **Which one of the following is NOT matched correctly?**
    A. Form of thought – loosening of association
    B. Content of thought – persecutory belief
    C. Stream of thought – poverty of speech
    D. Form of thought – obsessions
    E. Form of thought – circumstantiality

25. **Which one of the following is more common in manic rather than schizophrenic speech disturbance?**
    A. Clanging
    B. Derailment
    C. Thought blocking
    D. Tangentiality
    E. Poverty of content of speech

26. **A 66-year-old man tends to repeat the same answer for all subsequent questions. This is pathognomonic of**
    A. Schizophrenia
    B. Organic brain damage
    C. Mixed affective state
    D. Conversion disorder
    E. Stuttering

27. **Obsessions are intrusive and repetitive mental phenomenon. In which of the following forms can an obsession occur?**

    A. Thoughts
    B. Words
    C. Images
    D. Impulses
    E. All of the above

28. **Obsessions are appreciated to be against values and ideals of self. Which of the following terms corresponds to this description?**

    A. Ego-dystonic
    B. Ego-syntonic
    C. Ego-ideal
    D. Ego-neutral
    E. Ego-ridden

29. **Passivity phenomena can occur as any of the following EXCEPT**

    A. Thought insertion
    B. Thought withdrawal
    C. Thought broadcasting
    D. Thought blocking
    E. None of the above

30. **Which of the following is NOT a first-rank symptom of schizophrenia?**

    A. Thought echo
    B. Somatic hallucinations
    C. Delusional perception
    D. Thought withdrawal
    E. Made volition

31. **Which of the following statements with regard to first-rank symptoms is incorrect?**

    A. It is a comprehensive list of schizophrenic symptoms
    B. It emphasizes form not content
    C. It has clearly identifiable features
    D. They are seen more often in schizophrenia than other psychosis
    E. They are not essential for diagnosis

32. **A patient suffers from an osteoarthritic knee pain, but he believes it is caused by 'the leader of a cybernetic extermination gang' in an attempt to robotize him. Which of the following symptoms is he exhibiting?**

    A. Somatic hallucination
    B. Somatic passivity
    C. Somatization
    D. Body image disturbance
    E. Delusional perception

33. **Various dimensions of delusional experience include all EXCEPT**
    A. Distress
    B. Loss of insight
    C. Preoccupation
    D. Conviction
    E. Callousness

34. **Which of the following is NOT a primary delusion?**
    A. Delusional mood
    B. Delusional memory
    C. Delusional perception
    D. Delusional intuitions
    E. Delusional misinterpretation

35. **A 44-year-old man is taken into police custody for harassing his wife. He is convinced that she is having an affair but in fact, she isn't. Which of the following disorders cannot explain the above presentation?**
    A. Alcohol dependence
    B. Misidentification syndrome
    C. Delusional disorder
    D. Schizophrenia
    E. Dementia

36. **A 65-year-old woman believes that she is already dead. Similar delusions are reported in which of the following diseases?**
    A. Schizophrenia
    B. Depressive psychosis
    C. Late-onset depression
    D. Organic disorders
    E. All of the above

37. **Mr Spencer is a loving and caring husband of Martha. When Martha is pregnant, Mr Spencer develops symptoms of bloating, pelvic pain, and morning sickness. The main psychopathology in the above presentation is**
    A. A conversion symptom
    B. Delusion
    C. Hypochondriasis
    D. Body image disturbance
    E. Hallucination

38. **A 72-year-old lady complains of being infested with body lice. Her dermatologist could not find any signs of infestation but she insists that she could feel the lice moving on her skin and brings a matchbox full of skin scrapings for examination. Which of the following descriptions is most appropriate?**
    A. Obsession of contamination
    B. Compulsive skin picking
    C. Factitious dermatitis
    D. Somatization
    E. Ekbom's syndrome

39. **Which of the following is not a delusional misidentification?**
    A. Reduplicative paramnesia
    B. Cotard's syndrome
    C. Capgras' syndrome
    D. Fregoli's syndrome
    E. Intermetamorphosis

40. **Which of the following is FALSE with respect to Doppelganger?**
    A. It is an ideational rather than a perceptual disturbance
    B. It is known as double phenomenon
    C. It can occur in the absence of mental illness.
    D. It is a delusion of misidentification
    E. None of the above

41. **A patient feels very anxious leaving home. He feels people in the street are watching him and feels very self-conscious about what he does. He tries to interpret different gestures he could see others making in his presence. Which one of the following suits this description best?**
    A. Sensitive ideas of reference
    B. Agoraphobia
    C. Delusions of persecution
    D. Specific phobia
    E. Delusions of reference

42. **Overvalued ideas are NOT noted in the core symptoms of which one of the following disorders?**
    A. Body dysmorphic disorder
    B. Anorexia nervosa
    C. Morbid jealousy
    D. Trans-sexualism
    E. PTSD

43. **Which one of the following is not a type of normal thinking process?**

    A. Autistic thinking
    B. Dereistic thinking
    C. Fantasy thinking
    D. Rational thinking
    E. Desultory thinking

44. **In formal thought disorder, asyndesis refers to which of the following?**

    A. Lack of genuine causal links in speech
    B. Lack of information in speech
    C. Lack of logical arguments in speech
    D. Lack of wide vocabulary in speech
    E. Lack of adjectives in speech

45. **A patient who has taken lithium for some months discontinues it and says 'the ocean needs a sail as rat needs a tail, so write your exam and don't fail, results will be out in a mail'. Which of the following symptoms is he exhibiting?**

    A. Rhyming
    B. Punning
    C. Neologisms
    D. Pressured speech
    E. Metonymy

46. **Analyse the following speech sample and choose the appropriate description. 'The *whirl* of Susan's life, it's me... and I want to *whirl* happily. Stop all medicine, I will get more *whirl* every night. No doctor has the *whirl* to help...always liars...This *whirl* is full of mad people.'**

    A. Metonymy
    B. Neologism
    C. Verbigeration
    D. Paraphasia
    E. Stock word

47. **Which of the following psychopathological features could be diagnosed using sorting tests?**

    A. Overinclusion
    B. Verbigeration
    C. Echolalia
    D. Acalculia
    E. Anosognosia

48. **Analyse the following speech sample and choose appropriate description.**
    'Q: How many legs does a dog have? A: Five. Q: What comes after Saturday?
    A: Tuesday.'
    A. Vorbeireden
    B. Mitgehen
    C. Tangentiality
    D. Circumstantiality
    E. Stock words

49. **Which of the following is associated with circumstantiality?**
    A. Figure ground failure
    B. Affective changes
    C. Malingering
    D. Filling memory gaps
    E. None of the above

50. **In pure word deafness, which one of the following is impaired?**
    A. Reading
    B. Writing
    C. Speaking
    D. Comprehension
    E. Source localization

51. **Goldstein is associated with which of the following modes of thinking?**
    A. Desultory thinking
    B. Over inclusive thinking
    C. Illogical thinking
    D. Concrete thinking
    E. All of the above

52. **Bannister repertory grid can be used to measure which of the following**
    phenomena?
    A. Poverty of thought
    B. Psychomotor retardation
    C. Formal thought disorder
    D. Lack of empathy
    E. Lack of imagination

53. **Which of the following can be used to assess formal thought disorder in**
    schizophrenia?
    A. Cloze procedure
    B. Type–token ratio
    C. Word association tests
    D. Cohesion analysis
    E. All of the above

54. **Which of the following is a psychopathology of familiarity?**
   A. Déjà vu
   B. Confabulation
   C. Pseudologia
   D. Parapraxis
   E. Paraphasia

55. **Which one of the following is described as a core symptom of Ganser's syndrome?**
   A. Pseudohallucinations
   B. Approximate answers
   C. Somatic symptoms
   D. Indifference
   E. Lack of remorse

56. **Loss of insight is a common feature in schizophrenia. Which of the following neurological symptoms is comparable to loss of insight?**
   A. Object agnosia
   B. Simultagnosia
   C. Anosognosia
   D. Amnesia
   E. Apraxia

57. **Patients that complain of unusual symptoms, using the words 'as if', are most likely to have which of the following phenomena?**
   A. Déjà vu
   B. Jamais vu
   C. Depersonalization
   D. Formication
   E. Rumination

58. **A 43-year-old widow presents to the clinic with vague complaints. She is unable to express her emotions verbally. Difficulty in differentiating bodily sensation from emotional state is characteristic of patients with which of the following?**
   A. First-rank symptoms
   B. Loss of insight
   C. Frontal lesions
   D. Somatization
   E. Alcohol dependence

59. **Pathological gambling is considered as a part of which of the following cluster of symptoms?**

    A. Malingering
    B. Overvalued ideas
    C. Impulse control symptoms
    D. Manic symptoms
    E. Antisocial traits

60. **A 43-year-old widow presents to the clinic with vague complaints. She is unable to express her emotions verbally. Which of the following symptoms is LEAST likely to be seen in this lady?**

    A. Diminution of fantasy
    B. Reduced symbolic thinking
    C. Literal thinking concerned with details
    D. Difficulties in recognizing ones own feelings
    E. Amnesia for traumatic events in the past

61. **Near death experiences are related to which of the following phenomenology?**

    A. Passivity
    B. Possession
    C. Autoscopy
    D. Alienation
    E. Reincarnation

62. **Mutism is a catatonic sign. Which of the following with regard to mutism is true?**

    A. Patient can speak but not coherently
    B. Patient can comprehend but cannot speak
    C. Patient can make non-verbal sounds to communicate
    D. Patient cannot move her vocalizing muscles
    E. Patient can neither comprehend nor speak

63. **Astasia–abasia is associated with which one of the following disorders?**

    A. Multiple sclerosis
    B. Motor neurone disease
    C. Sarcoidosis
    D. Dissociation disorder
    E. Delusional disorder

64. **Which one of the following patients CANNOT experience hallucinations?**

    A. 12-year-old boy with no mental illness
    B. 34-year-old man with IQ of 45
    C. 23-year-old man who is deaf and mute
    D. 47-year-old lady with bilateral acoustic neuroma
    E. None of the above

65. **A 32-year-old carpenter starts believing that his new laptop is sending him infrared signals. Which of the following processes CANNOT explain the development of the above belief?**

A. Jumping to conclusions
B. Theory of mind defect
C. Attributional bias
D. Defective probabilistic reasoning
E. Subvocal motor activation

66. **Which of the following is considered to be the most important difference between primary and secondary delusions?**

A. Preceding mental phenomenon
B. Time of onset
C. Associated distress
D. Degree of impairment
E. None of the above

67. **A 65-year-old housewife is admitted to a hospital in Durham following a head injury. She claims that the same hospital has an extension that runs into Dundee, and she could be in Dundee at the same time as she is in Durham. Which of the following entities should be considered in her presentation?**

A. Schizophrenia
B. Delusional disorder
C. Reduplicative paramnesia
D. Dementia
E. Multiple personality disorder

68. **Disorientation of age seen in schizophrenia is more common in which of the following patient groups?**

A. Acute episode
B. Younger age
C. Female patients
D. Chronic schizophrenia
E. Associated delirium

69. **Double orientation is a phenomenon seen in chronic schizophrenia. It refers to which of the following?**

A. Visual splitting
B. Oriented to time but not place and person
C. Having delusional orientation separate from reality
D. Intermingled delusional and real life orientation
E. None of the above

pharmacist has asked you to reduce or change antipsychotic
prescriptions to an inpatient as he has developed akathisia. Akathisia refers
to which of the following descriptions?

A. Poor attention span
B. Recurrent violent impulses
C. Restlessness without autonomic features
D. Anxiety characterized by cognitive and somatic features
E. Fidgety, shuffling gait

71. **Which of the following is not a catatonic symptom?**

A. Posturing
B. Negativism
C. Ambitendence
D. Astasia–abasia
E. Mitgehen

72. **Which of the following statements accurately differentiates catatonic rigidity from neurological spasticity?**

A. Tone normalizes for voluntary acts in catatonia
B. Tremors are superimposed in spasticity
C. Catatonia is generalized not specific to a muscle group
D. Small muscles are not affected by catatonia
E. Catatonia disappears while sleeping

73. **Which of the following differentiates the anhedonia seen in depression versus anhedonia seen in chronic schizophrenia? Anhedonia differs in**

A. Quality
B. Severity
C. Mode of onset
D. Chronicity
E. Insight

74. **Folie a deux is characterized by which of the following clinical descriptions?**

A. Two persons having the same diagnosis
B. Twins having the same psychotic illness
C. Two persons sharing delusional content
D. Two delusions with the same theme
E. Two delusions seen at the same time

75. **Which of the following pair is correctly matched?**

A. Obsessions – ego dystonic
B. Delusions – ego dystonic
C. Over valued ideas – ego dystonic
D. Confabulation – ego dystonic
E. All of the above

76. **A patient suffering from schizophrenia makes up a totally new word that is not in a dictionary – 'tynmis' for sausage. Which of the following phenomena is he exhibiting?**
    A. Metonymy
    B. Neologism
    C. Verbigeration
    D. Paraphasia
    E. Stock word

77. **Which of the following describes the most common type of hypnogogic hallucinations?**
    A. Being called by name
    B. Seeing dead persons
    C. Seeing monsters
    D. Derogatory comments
    E. Musical sound

78. **Which of the following is a neurological illness that mimics schizophrenic speech disturbance?**
    A. Broca's aphasia
    B. Alexia with agraphia
    C. Wernicke's aphasia
    D. Transcortical aphasia
    E. Astereognosia

79. **Which of the following is not a type of paranoid delusion?**
    A. 'Someone is following me.'
    B. 'People in the street are talking about me.'
    C. 'Aliens are making my body rot.'
    D. 'The Messiah is watching my every move.'
    E. 'Martians have landed on earth.'

80. **A patient with dementia is asked to perform a cognitive task beyond his current ability. He becomes very agitated. This is called**
    A. Catastrophic reaction
    B. Temper tantrum
    C. Confabulation
    D. Denial
    E. Magnification

81. **A 23-year-old man points to his left elbow and says he could hear voices coming from it. Which of the following symptoms is he exhibiting?**
    A. Anosognosia
    B. Somatic hallucination
    C. Extracampine hallucination
    D. Auditory hallucination
    E. Somatization

82. **Which of the following symptoms denotes an abnormal psychopathology whenever present?**
    A. Obsessions
    B. Delusions
    C. Hallucinations
    D. Depersonalization
    E. Amnesia

83. **When a patient is asked where she is living, she says 'Helltown' instead of 'Hilton'. She quickly corrects her error after saying the word. This is an example of which of the following phenomena?**
    A. Parapraxis
    B. Confabulation
    C. Pseudologia fantastica
    D. Manipulation
    E. Impulsivity

84. **Pronominal reversal is a symptom associated with which of the following disorders?**
    A. Schizophrenia
    B. Conduction aphasia
    C. Pseudobulbar dysarthria
    D. Autism
    E. Mania

85. **Which of the following refers to the sign present in autistic children who continually rotate in the direction in which their head is turned?**
    A. Vertigo
    B. Automatic obedience
    C. Catalepsy
    D. Twirling
    E. Twisting

1. B.   Psychopathology is the systematic study of abnormal experience, cognition, and behaviour. It consists of two major divisions –

1. explanatory psychopathology, which attempts to explain causative factors through theory generation or experimental construction; hence explanatory psychopathology includes experimental (e.g. behaviourism) and theoretical (e.g. psychoanalysis) subtypes;
2. descriptive psychopathology, which precisely describes and categorizes abnormal experiences as reported by the patient and observed from his behaviour.

Sims A. *Symptom in the Mind*, 3rd edn. London: Elsevier Science, 2003, p. 2.

2. B.   This patient is exhibiting a catatonic symptom called negativism. Patients with negativism resist or oppose all passive movements attempted by the examiner. A mild form of such resistance is called *Gegenhalten* or opposition. In extreme forms it is called negativism, where apparently motiveless resistance to all interference is found. Negativism can be a frustrating symptom, especially for carers involved in offering nursing assistance to the patient. The catatonic symptom of blocking or obstruction (or *Sperrung*) refers to a phenomenon similar to thought blocking but occurs while carrying out motor acts. A patient with obstruction suddenly stops a motor act for no reason, without any warning. This may be demonstrated by asking the patient to move a part of his body; the movement is generally well begun, but then stops halfway without any indication. In ambitendency the patient makes a series of tentative, opposing, alternate movements that do not reach the intended goal. This becomes evident when the patient is asked to carry out a motor act, for example asking the patient to show his tongue will elicit repeated protrusion and retraction of tongue as if the patient is undecided about showing his tongue.

Sims A. *Symptom in the Mind*, 3rd edn. London: Elsevier Science, 2003, p. 365.

3. A.   While humour may facilitate the process of clinical interview on certain occasions, it is not a necessary component of descriptive psychopathology. There are two essential components of descriptive psychopathology: (1) the observation of behaviour; and (2) the empathic assessment of subjective experience. The latter was referred to by Jaspers as phenomenology and implies that the patient is able to introspect and describe his internal experiences and the doctor recognizes and understands the description. To describe a phenomenon, it is important to appreciate the phenomenon from the beholder's point of view. This attempt to 'feel like how your patient might feel' is very different from feeling sorry or pity for your patient. The former is called empathy while the latter is called sympathy. Empathy is an essential component to learn further about the pathological processes taking place in a patient.

Sims A. *Symptom in the Mind*, 3rd edn. London: Elsevier Science, 2003, pp. 5, 10.

4. D. The patient usually presents with loss or impairment of functions, the reasons for which will reveal the contents of the patient's thoughts and feelings. Form is the technical term (e.g. phobia, obsession, or delusion) used to identify a recurring pattern of experience or behaviour and so helps in diagnosing the psychiatric disorder. Content is essential for decisions about the management of the patient and family (suicidal content, admission, etc.), and is an important aspect of the severity of the disorder. A symptom described using descriptive psychopathology has both form and content as equally important components. The same content can occur in different forms, for example the content 'I'm too fat' can occur as an obsession, delusion, overvalued idea, or even hallucination.

Sims A. *Symptom in the Mind*, 3rd edn. London: Elsevier Science, 2003, p. 16.

5. E. Stimulus may be perceived as corresponding object but not as accurate as the real object. This is a perceptual error (sensory distortion), and can be associated with changes in physical properties, for example size, shape, intensity, and colour. In depression and hypoactive delirium there is dulled perception. Intense perceptions can occur in mania, hyperactive delirium, and drug-induced states (hallucinogens). Hyperacusis is especially seen in migraine and alcohol hangover.

Sims A. *Symptom in the Mind*, 3rd edn. London: Elsevier Science, 2003, p. 94.

6. A. A perceptual error associated with changes in shape of objects, especially with loss of symmetry, is called dysmegalopsia. The objects can shrink in size (micropsia) or enlarge (macropsia). These are usually organic and could be related to ictal (parietal) or ocular pathology (accommodation errors – paralysed accommodation can cause micropsia). They are also rarely seen in acute schizophrenia. Hallucinogens (e.g. mescaline) can also change the colour of perceived objects or make components of an object (e.g. body parts) be seen detached in space.

Sims A. *Symptom in the Mind*, 3rd edn. London: Elsevier Science, 2003, p. 94.

7. B. Imagery is not a perception because there is no stimulus involved and no object perceived; it is essentially a fantasy. Imagery refers to images produced voluntarily with complete insight that they are a mental phenomena and not of external origin. Imageries lack the 'objective' quality of hallucinations and normal sense perceptions.

Sims A. *Symptom in the Mind*, 3rd edn. London: Elsevier Science, 2003, p. 92.

8. D. There are three major types of illusions: in affect illusion the prevailing emotional state leads to misperceptions, for example a depressed patient reading 'deed' as 'dead', a boy frightened of the dark seeing monsters from innocuous shadows. Pareidolia refers to perceiving formed objects from ambiguous stimuli, for example seeing cars in the clouds. It is common in delirium, especially in children. They are often playful – not characteristic of any psychotic illness. Completion illusion is due to inattention; stimulus that does not form a complete object might be perceived to be complete, for example CCOK is read as COOK. Eidetic imagery is considered to be a special ability of memory wherein visual images are drawn from memory accurately, at will and described as if being perceived currently. This is not a perceptual distortion but closely linked to mental imagery and it is often noted in children.

Sims A. *Symptom in the Mind*, 3rd edn. London: Elsevier Science, 2003, p. 97.

9.A. Pareidolia refers to perceiving formed objects from ambiguous stimuli, for example seeing faces in a fire or hidden messages when records are played in reverse. It is coloured by prevailing emotion and not entirely due to inattention or affective change; fantasy and imagery play a part in addition to actual sense perception. On paying extra effort the object intensifies and does not disappear. Pareidolia is common in febrile delirium, especially in children, and also in hallucinogen use. They are under voluntary control and often playful. Occurrence of pareidolia is not characteristic of any psychotic illness.

Sims A. *Symptom in the Mind*, 3rd edn. London: Elsevier Science, 2003, p. 97.

10. D. Hallucinations have several important qualities which are essential in differentiating them from other mental phenomena. Hallucinations take place at the same time and in the same space as other perceptions, for example 'an angel is standing in the corner of my room'. This is different from fantasy or imagery which takes place in a subjective space. They are experienced as sensations – not as thoughts – in contrast to obsessional images. The percept has all the qualities of a real world object , that is a patient when hallucinating believes that the percept can be experienced in other modalities too, like a real object which can be seen, felt, smelt, and heard. Pseudohallucinations are defined variously. The term is used to describe hallucination-like experiences with retained insight (so it is not sought in other modalities of perception). It is also used to describe hallucination-like experiences that take place in a subjective space, for example 'a voice inside my head'.

Sims A. *Symptom in the Mind*, 3rd edn. London: Elsevier Science, 2003, p. 99.

11.A. Elementary hallucinations are unstructured hallucinations that are seen in acute organic states. They are composed of sounds or flashes without being fully formed. Elementary hallucinations can precede development of fully formed hallucinations, especially in alcoholic hallucinosis. The flashes of lights are also called phosphenes. Words such as 'go' are meaningful and so cannot be a part of elementary hallucination.

Sims A. *Symptom in the Mind*, 3rd edn. London: Elsevier Science, 2003, p. 100.

12. D. Phonemes are any auditory hallucinations that occur as human voices. Schizophrenic phonemes are usually multiple voices. The voices may or may not be recognizable. These voices are usually male with a different accent but speaking in one's mother tongue. Schizophrenic hallucinations are usually episodic – almost never continuous. Continuous, non-stop hallucinations should make one suspect the veracity of the reported experience.

Sims A. *Symptom in the Mind*, 3rd edn. London: Elsevier Science, 2003, p. 100.

13. E. Occipital lobe tumours, postconcussional states, epileptic twilight state, hepatic failure (any toxic delirium), and dementia are some of the known causes of visual hallucinations. In fact, nearly 30% of old-age psychiatric referrals have visual hallucinations. Solvent sniffing and hallucinogens can cause elementary visual hallucinations such as light flashes. In dementia of Lewy body type visual hallucinations are a prominent feature.

Sims A. *Symptom in the Mind*, 3rd edn. London: Elsevier Science, 2003, p. 103.

14. A. Elderly patients having normal consciousness and no brain pathology but with reduced visual acuity due to ocular problems experience vivid, distinct, usually well-coloured hallucinations. This is known by the eponym Charles Bonnet syndrome. Paradoxically these perceptions are clear and colourful in contrast to real sensation, which is blurred due to eye disease. These hallucinations are mostly in the form of humans, or at times animals and cartoons. These objects usually show movement, and can be voluntarily controlled to an extent as they disappear on closing the eyes. Insight about unreality is usually preserved – though they may evoke emotions, including fear and joy. About one-third of Charles Bonnet hallucinations are elementary, unformed hallucinations. Usually these hallucinations are located in external space.

Sims A. *Symptom in the Mind*, 3rd edn. London: Elsevier Science, 2003, p. 104.

15. C. Lilliputian hallucinations can occur in visual or haptic mode – they usually involve seeing tiny people or animals (or feeling diminutive insects crawling if haptic) and are seen in delirium tremens. Unlike other organic visual hallucinations, lilliputian hallucinations can be accompanied by pleasure (though this is often intermingled with terror). These are not the same as micropsia. Micropsia is a perceptual distortion but not a hallucination as there is a stimulus which is perceived to be erroneously small. Perception of small objects in the absence of such stimuli is a lilliputian hallucination.

Sims A. *Symptom in the Mind*, 3rd edn. London: Elsevier Science, 2003, p. 105.

16. B. Palinopsia (*palin* for 'again' and *opsia* for 'seeing'). is a visual disturbance that causes images to persist even after their corresponding stimulus has ceased. It is seen in LSD use, migraine, occipital epilepsy, and head trauma. It is similar to afterimage but colour inversion (usually shadows or distorted colours) noted in afterimages is conspicuously absent. Formication (formic acid – from ants) is a special type of haptic hallucination. It is often an unpleasant sensation of little animals or insects crawling under the skin, seen in delirium tremens and cocaine intoxication.

Smith, P et al. Palinopsia. The Lancet, 361, 1098–1098

17. C. Autoscopic hallucinations are the visual experience of seeing oneself. It is seen predominantly in males compared to females at a ratio of 2:1. Impaired consciousness is a common accompaniment and depression is the commonest psychiatric cause of autoscopy. They are also called phantom mirror images and may take the form of pseudohallucinations. Schizophrenia (where autoscopic experience is usually pseudohallucinatory), TLE, and parietal lesions (organic states more likely to have true hallucinations) are also implicated. In negative autoscopy one looks into a mirror and sees no image at all.

Sims A. *Symptom in the Mind*, 3rd edn. London: Elsevier Science, 2003, p. 105.

18. D. Chronic benzodiazepine use leads to the development of dependence, with a characteristic withdrawal syndrome that presents with anxiety and agitation, insomnia, tremor, depersonalization, and, if severe, can lead to seizures and delirium. Kinaesthetic or proprioceptive hallucinations refer to joint or muscle sense, often linked to bizarre somatic delusions. Kinaesthetic hallucinations are seen in benzodiazepine withdrawal and alcohol intoxication.

Sims A. *Symptom in the Mind*, 3rd edn. London: Elsevier Science, 2003, p. 106.

19. C. The common experience of phantom limb is a body image disturbance and not a hallucination; though it is in external space, it does not satisfy other qualities of hallucination and patients are usually aware of unreality. It is a body image disturbance with a neurological basis.

Sims A. *Symptom in the Mind*, 3rd edn. London: Elsevier Science, 2003, p. 266.

20. A.   Extracampine hallucinations are hallucinations that occur outside the normal field of perception, for example images seen behind your back, under your sternum, or hearing voices from Inverness, etc. (if you are not living in Inverness, of course!). They occur in schizophrenia, epilepsy, and also in hypnagogic hallucinations of healthy people – so they are not diagnostically important.

Sims A. *Symptom in the Mind*, 3rd edn. London: Elsevier Science, 2003, p. 112.

21. C.   In functional hallucinations an external stimulus provokes a hallucination, and both hallucination and stimulus are in same modality but individually perceived, for example voices heard simultaneously when ever the noise of water running through a kitchen tap is heard. They are not illusions, as the stimulus is perceived appropriately (noise of water), but in addition there is another perception (voices) without an appropriate object. If hallucinations in one modality are provoked reflexively by stimulus in another modality, for example seeing an angel when ever listening to music, then this is called reflex hallucination. The phenomenon of perceiving a stimulus of one modality in a different modality (may be single or multiple modalities) is called synaesthesia, for example tasting the music, hearing colours, and smelling voices.

Sims A. *Symptom in the Mind*, 3rd edn. London: Elsevier Science, 2003, p. 112

22. B.   Synaesthesia is defined broadly as a mingling of the senses. People with the condition may see a colour when they look at a number or hear a tone when they see a colour. It is not a hallucination as the perception comes from an appropriate stimulus. The original stimulus is simultaneously perceived in appropriate modality in addition to the cross modality perception (*syn* – joint, simultaneous).

Sims A. *Symptom in the Mind*, 3rd edn. London: Elsevier Science, 2003, p. 113
Ramachandran VS and Hubbard EM. Synaesthesia: A window into perception, thought and language. *Journal of Consciousness Studies* 2001; **8**: 3–34.

23. E.   Synaesthesia is common in females (4:1), runs in families, and colour–number synaesthesia is the most common form. It is thought to be due to extensive cross-wiring between multimodal association regions in some people, probably due to failed selective pruning. It is not a hallucination.

Baron-Cohen S, Burt L, Smith-Laittan F, *et al.* Synaesthesia: prevalence and familiality. *Perception* 1996; **25**: 1073–1079.

24. D.   The pathology of thought can be divided into content (What is being 'thought about'?), form (In what manner (or shape) is the thought present?), and stream or flow (How is it being thought about?). Disordered thought content is seen as delusions, for example persecutory themes, obsessions, or preoccupations. Overvalued idea is also a disorder of thought content. Disordered stream of thought is seen as poverty of thought, pressure of speech, and crowding of thoughts. Disordered form of thought, as seen in schizophrenia and other psychotic disorders, refers to a set of various alterations in the thinking process – loosening of associations, metonyms, tangentiality, and circumstantiality to name a few. As an analogy, 'thought' can be considered to be a box of packed fruits bought in the supermarket. Form is equivalent to the shape of the box (e.g. rectangular plastic box), content is equivalent to the type of fruit (e.g. oranges or peaches) and stream is equivalent to the number of fruits in the box (e.g. 6 or 12).

Sims A. *Symptom in the Mind*, 3rd edn. London: Elsevier Science, 2003, p. 149.

25. A. Of all thought disorders classified by Andreasen, clanging and flight are more common in mania while derailment (loosening) and thought blocking (and to some extent tangentiality and poverty of content of speech) are seen often in schizophrenia – other items were not thought to be specific for a particular psychiatric condition.

Andreasen, N. C. (1979) Thought, language, and communication disorders: I. Clinical assessment, definition of terms, and evaluation of their reliability. Archives of General Psychiatry, 36, 1315–1321

26. B. In perseveration the thought process tends to persist beyond a point at which they are relevant. Perseveration generally occurs with clouded consciousness and is considered pathognomonic of organic brain disease. Perseveration can be demonstrated verbally or through repetitive motor activity. It can be seen in schizophrenia too. Stuttering is due to motor speech in-coordination and does not involve the mechanism of perseveration.

Sims A. *Symptom in the Mind*, 3rd edn. London: Elsevier Science, 2003, pp. 69, 157.

27. E. Obsessions usually evoke distress and anxiety and are not pleasurable by definition. They are unwanted, intrusive, repetitive, senseless thoughts experienced by patients as troublesome and resisted. Obsessions can be thoughts, words, impulses, or images. They usually occur in themes of sex, religion, violence, safety, and grooming (e.g. orderliness, washing out germs, etc.).

Sims A. *Symptom in the Mind*, 3rd edn. London: Elsevier Science, 2003, p. 336.

28. A. In obsessions, though the appearance of the thoughts themselves is appreciated to be beyond a patient's control, they are not claimed to be due to an external agency. Obsessions are regarded to be one's own mind's product but ego-dystonic – against one's values and needs. Often during the course of OCD, primary obsessions fade while compulsions dominate the clinical picture; some compulsions can be mental behaviours such as praying, counting, etc.

Sims A. *Symptom in the Mind*, 3rd edn. London: Elsevier Science, 2003, p. 338.

29. D. A subjective disturbance in thinking seen in schizophrenia is described as passivity, which can occur in the form of thought insertion, thought withdrawal, and thought broadcasting. These are first-rank symptoms of schizophrenia. Thought blocking is not a passivity or alienation phenomenon.

Simon M and Spence SA. Re-examining thought insertion: Semi-structured literature review and conceptual analysis. *British Journal of Psychiatry* 2003; **182**: 293–298.

30. B. The first-rank symptoms are:

Three hallucinations:

Audible thoughts (thought echo)
Voices heard arguing (3rd person)
Voices heard commenting on one's actions (running commentary)

Three 'made' phenomena:

Made affect (someone controlling the mood/ affect)
Made volition (someone controlling the action – usually a completed act)
Made impulse (someone controlling the desire to act – not completed act but the drive. If the action has been carried out, then the patient admits to ownership of the act, not the impulse behind it)

Three thought phenomena: (experiences themselves are more important than later explanations of how a patient interprets them)

Thought withdrawal
Thought insertion (external agency inserting thoughts into the patient)
Thought broadcast (also called thought diffusion – as if in a television broadcast, everyone comes to know about the patient's thinking as and when the patient thinks – refers to loss of privacy of thoughts. Contrast with referential delusion – 'people act as if they know what I am thinking')

Two isolated symptoms:

Delusional perception
Experience of sensations on the body caused by external agency (somatic passivity)

Somatic hallucinations are NOT first rank symptoms unless there is a delusional elaboration and attribution of the origin of sensations to an external agency (passivity).

Sims A. *Symptom in the Mind*, 3rd edn. London: Elsevier Science, 2003, p. 165.

31. A. Kurt Schneider proposed an empirical cluster of symptoms, one or more of which, in the absence of evidence of organic processes, can be used as positive evidence for schizophrenia. These symptoms are not comprehensive features of schizophrenia; they are clearly identifiable, frequently occurring, and occur more often in schizophrenia than any other disorder. First-rank symptoms emphasize form rather than content, for example the fact that one's thoughts are heard as echo of voices is more important than the actual content of the voices; this increases cross-cultural reliability, although variations exist. First-rank symptoms have some diagnostic but no prognostic importance in schizophrenia.

Sims A. *Symptom in the Mind*, 3rd edn. London: Elsevier Science, 2003, p. 166.

32. B. Somatic passivity refers to experience of sensations in one's body believed to be caused by some external agency. It can follow a normal sensation, such an osteoarthritic knee pain, ascribed to be caused by an external agency, as in this case.

Sims A. *Symptom in the Mind*, 3rd edn. London: Elsevier Science, 2003, p. 169.

33. E. Kendler (1983) has listed the dimensions of delusional experiences (also incorporated in the Maudsley Assessment of Delusions Scale) – conviction, extension (to various spheres of life), disorganization (or organization–internal consistency and systematization), bizarreness (especially in schizophrenia), and pressure (includes preoccupation and distress). Acting on delusion, seeking evidence, and lack of insight can be added as other qualities. These various dimensions exist in a continuum with normal beliefs.

Sims A. *Symptom in the Mind*, 3rd edn. London: Elsevier Science, 2003, p. 119.
Kendler KS, Glazer W, Morgenstern H. Dimensions of delusional experience. *American Journal of Psychiatry* 1983; **140**: 466–469.

34. E. Primary delusions are defined in two different ways: (1) Jaspers' concept of primary delusions is that they are un-understandable and cannot be reduced further to any other mental experiences; and (2) primary delusions are also thought of as the first abnormal mental experience to occur in schizophrenia prodrome (primary as per temporal sequence). Often both of these are true – primary delusions are not only irreducible but also precede other mental phenomena. The four types of primary delusions are: (1) delusional mood; (2) delusional perception; (3) delusional memory; and (4) autochthonous delusion (often simply referred to as a primary delusion).

Sims A. *Symptom in the Mind*, 3rd edn. London: Elsevier Science, 2003, p. 120.

35. B. Morbid jealousy can occur in various forms – delusion, overvalued idea, in depression, and in anxiety states; it is not a misidentification syndrome. It was first described by Ey. It is common in alcoholics. It has a potential for violence, especially against the perceived rival for one's partner, and can occur among cohabitants and homosexual couples too.

Sims A. *Symptom in the Mind*, 3rd edn. London: Elsevier Science, 2003, p. 132.

36. E. Cotard's syndrome is severe depression with nihilistic and hypochondriacal delusions tinged with grandiosity and a negative attitude. It is not related to delusional misidentification. Cotard's syndrome is seen in schizophrenia, though more commonly in depressive psychosis. It is generally seen in elderly people and is also reported in organic lesions and migraine.

Sims A. *Symptom in the Mind*, 3rd edn. London: Elsevier Science, 2003, p. 13.

37. A. Couvade syndrome describes a sympathetic pregnancy that affects husbands (rarely other family members) during their wives' pregnancies. It is most frequent between 3 and 9 months of a spouse's pregnancy. It is a conversion symptom and not delusional as the husband does not believe he is pregnant! Pseudocyesis is a condition where a woman experiences clinical signs of pregnancy without being pregnant, and she may become fully convinced of being pregnant.

Sims A. *Symptom in the Mind*, 3rd edn. London: Elsevier Science, 2003, p. 288.

38. E. Delusional infestation (Ekbom's syndrome) is a delusion of parasitic (macroscopic) infestation with classical matchbox sign. An old lady comes to clinic with a match box of skin scrapings, as evidence for the parasite that infests her, causing itching. This can predate the onset of dementia. It may or may not be associated with a somatic tactile hallucination. It is not the same as compulsive skin picking, where the psychopathology is one of compulsion and not delusion. In factitious dermatitis, patients seek medical attention without obvious monetary gain in order to be in a patient role. They induce skin lesions using chemicals or medicinal products in order to 'become a patient'. This lady is not having somatization where multiple, non-specific somatic (mostly pain) symptoms are present.

Sims A. *Symptom in the Mind*, 3rd edn. London: Elsevier Science, 2003, p. 139.

39. B. The various misidentification syndromes are: (1) Capgras syndrome, where a patient believes that a person, usually close to him, has been replaced by an exact double; (2) Fregoli syndrome, where there is false identification of strangers as familiar persons; a familiar person is thought to be taking various disguises; (3) syndrome of subjective doubles, where the patient believes that another person has been physically transformed into his own self and the patient is convinced that exact doubles of him- or herself exist; and (4) intermetamorphosis – Person A becomes C, C becomes B, etc.; people keep transforming their physical and psychological identities.

Sims A. *Symptom in the Mind*, 3rd edn. London: Elsevier Science, 2003, p. 134.

40. D.   Doppelganger is also known as double phenomenon – it is the awareness of one's existence as being both outside and inside oneself. It is cognitive and ideational, as opposed to autoscopy which is perceptual. It can occur in the absence of mental illness too. It is not related to delusional misidentification syndromes where there is pathology of familiarity.

Sims A. *Symptom in the Mind*, 3rd edn. London: Elsevier Science, 2003, p. 217.

41. A.   Ideas of reference are seen in paranoid personality disorder where the individual is unduly self-conscious and feels that people take notice of him or observe things about him that he would rather not be seen. It can also precede development of full-blown schizophrenia, where it is called sensitive ideas of reference or 'sensitiver Beziehungswahn'.

Sims A. *Symptom in the Mind*, 3rd edn. London: Elsevier Science, 2003, p. 144.

42. E.   Overvalued ideas (Wernicke) are solitary, abnormal beliefs that are neither delusional nor obsessional in nature, but dominate a person's actions. They have a poor prognosis and tend to dominate the sufferer's life. Common conditions presenting with overvalued ideas are paranoid or anankastic personality disorder, Body dysmorphophobia, anorexia nervosa, morbid jealousy, and trans-sexualism.

Sims A. *Symptom in the Mind*, 3rd edn. London: Elsevier Science, 2003, p. 143; see Table 8.1, p. 144.

43. E.   Normal thinking is of three types (or functions): (1) Fantasy/ dereistic thinking or autistic thinking: There is no goal direction in the thoughts. The contents are often unrealistic, for example day dreaming. It is seen predominantly in cluster A personality, dissociation, and pseudologia fantastica. (2) Imaginative thinking: This includes fantasy elements but admixed with true memory and abstract concepts. Imaginative thinking is often goal directed and does not cross boundaries of possibility and realism. Determining tendency of thoughts are preserved, for example lateral thinking. (3) Rational or conceptual thinking: This is often based on material reality and uses logic. Desultory thinking is a type of formal thought disturbance proposed by Carl Schneider.

Sims A. *Symptom in the Mind*, 3rd edn. London: Elsevier Science, 2003, p. 150.

44. A.   Asyndesis is defined as lack of genuine causal links in speech. It is a type of formal thought disorder observed by Cameron. Poverty of content of speech or alogia is a term used to describe lack of information in speech. Lack of wide vocabulary could be measured by poor type–token ratio. Low type–token ratio has been observed in schizophrenia.

Sims A. *Symptom in the Mind*, 3rd edn. London: Elsevier Science, 2003, p. 160.

45. A.   In clang associations, thoughts are associated by the sound of words rather than their meaning, that is through rhymes (rail/ tail/ sail) or puns (one word with two meanings rose = flower/ past tense of rise). Clang associations can form the basis for flight of ideas. Pressured speech is not a formal thought disturbance; it is rather a disturbance in stream of thought.

Sims A. *Symptom in the Mind*, 3rd edn. London: Elsevier Science, 2003, p. 183.

46. E.   Neologism refers to making up a totally new word that is not in dictionary or using a known word with a completely different meaning, for example 'inkur' for pen (here a new word is created) or 'roast' for pen (here a known word is employed different to normal usage). Metonyms are word approximations, for example paperskate for pen. Stock words are either newly synthesized or already known words but used in an idiosyncratic way repeatedly, often with many meanings and in different contexts, sometimes dominating a discourse, as in this example. The word 'whirl' here stands for 'meaning', 'to live', 'to sleep', 'nature' etc. Neologisms, stock words, and metonyms together constitute private symbolism noted in schizophrenia.

Sims A. *Symptom in the Mind*, 3rd edn. London: Elsevier Science, 2003, pp. 175, 181.

47. A. In overinclusive thinking ideas that are only remotely related to the concept under consideration become incorporated in the patient's thinking. Normal conceptual boundaries are lost in overinclusive thinking. This is used to explain the thought disorders in schizophrenia and is different from the mechanism in flight of ideas. Sorting tests can be used to test overinclusion. It occurs in nearly 50% of schizophrenia patients, especially when they are acutely ill.

Sims A. *Symptom in the Mind*, 3rd edn. London: Elsevier Science, 2003, p. 160.

48. A. Vorbeireden ('talking past the point') is often used interchangeably with vorbeigehen ('going past the point'). Vorbeigehen was originally defined as part of the 'Ganser syndrome' whereby some criminals would give incorrect answers ('approximate answers') to simple questions. The incorrect answers themselves suggest that the question was well comprehended and the correct answer was known (e.g. Question: How many legs do dogs have? Answer: Five).

Sims A. *Symptom in the Mind*, 3rd edn. London: Elsevier Science, 2003, p. 173.

49. A. In circumstantiality, thinking proceeds slowly, with many unnecessary details and digressions, before returning to the point. It is seen in some patients with temporal lobe epilepsy or alcohol-induced persisting dementia, learning difficulty, and in obsessional personalities. It is a formal thought disorder where figure ground differentiation apparently fails. It is not due to affective changes such as mania. It is not the same as tangentiality – the patient never reaches the point in tangentiality, whereas they do reach the point in circumstantiality. Imagine a spiral that eventually touches its centre, while tangent scrapes through the edge and never reaches the centre. Circumstantiality may be related to loosened associations and usually develops within the setting of a delusional mood in schizophrenia; it may be due to an impairment of a central filtering process that normally inhibits external sensations and internal thoughts that are irrelevant to a given focus of attention.

Sims A. *Symptom in the Mind*, 3rd edn. London: Elsevier Science, 2003, p. 154.

50. D. In pure word deafness the patient can speak, read, and write fluently, but comprehension of speech is impaired. In pure word dumbness the disturbance is limited to an inability to produce and repeat words at will. In pure word blindness (alexia) speech and writing are normal but the patient cannot read. Comprehension of spoken words is preserved in pure word blindness.

Sims A. *Symptom in the Mind*, 3rd edn. London: Elsevier Science, 2003, p. 176.

51. D. Concrete thinking is seen as thinking characterized by a predominance of actual objects and events and the absence of concepts and generalizations, that is failed abstraction. It is recognizable clinically but difficult to measure using psychometric tests. According to Goldstein concrete thinking is a direct result of loss of abstract thinking. It is observed that concrete thinking is evident in speech-disordered (FTD) schizophrenia patients, but not in the non-FTD group (Allen 1984). It is also seen in frontotemporal dementia.

Sims A. *Symptom in the Mind*, 3rd edn. London: Elsevier Science, 2003, p. 181.
Allen HA. Positive and negative symptoms and the thematic organization of schizophrenic speech. *British Journal of Psychiatry* 1984; **144**: 611–617.

52. C. Schizophrenic thought disorder could be measured using repertory grids (Bannister) based on Kelly's personal construct theory. The patient is asked to score different elements (can be relatives or friends) under different constructs (qualities of them). Normally, one would expect congruence between different constructs scored for an element, for example Mum is helpful and she is also kind and supportive. But in schizophrenia the predictability of an element's quality using prior constructs is affected. (Mum is helpful but scores low on kindness and support offered). This is called serial invalidation and is more pronounced for peoples than objects, showing that thought disorder affects interpersonal realm more than other spheres. The scores can be used to draw a semantic space, demonstrating graphical connections between people and qualities in a patient's personal world.

Sims A. *Symptom in the Mind*, 3rd edn. London: Elsevier Science, 2003, p. 161; see Fig. 9.8.

53. E. All of these stated methods have been employed to quantify formal thought disorder seen in schizophrenia. Word association tests are abnormal in schizophrenia. Patients with schizophrenia prefer dominant meaning of a word, despite the context of its usage, for example court means 'law-room' not tennis court, in spite of a discussion about sports. This abnormality can be tested using word association tests. In cloze procedure parts of one's recorded speech are deleted to see if meaning could be still predicted; predictability was reduced in the speech of patients with schizophrenia. Type–token ratio refers to the ratio between the number of different words used during a discourse and the total number of spoken words. Impoverished vocabulary was noted with low type–token ratio among schizophrenia patients. Cohesion analysis refers to the analysis of links between sentences and words in a discourse. It shows that schizophrenia patients use less referential ties (e.g. using pronouns without mentioning a subject in first place) and more lexical ties (i.e. connected words).

Sims A. *Symptom in the Mind*, 3rd edn. London: Elsevier Science, 2003, p. 185.

54. A. Déjà vu is the feeling of having seen or experienced an event, which in fact is being experienced for the first time. Jamais vu is loss of familiarity of an event or situation that has been experienced before. Both can occur in normal people, and in temporal lobe epilepsy. Déjà vu and jamais vu are considered as pathologies of familiarity.

Sims A. *Symptom in the Mind*, 3rd edn. London: Elsevier Science, 2003, p. 84.

55. B. Ganser's syndrome includes:

Approximate answers
Clouding of consciousness with disorientation
Psychogenic physical symptoms – analgesia and hyperaesthesia
Pseudohallucinations (not always present)
Patients with Ganser's syndrome may be amnesic for their abnormal behaviour.

Sims A. *Symptom in the Mind*, 3rd edn. London: Elsevier Science, 2003, p. 252.

56. C. Insight is a multidimensional concept; it is not useful to restrict oneself to the assessment of 'presence' or 'absence' of insight. Though traditionally insight was considered to be present in those with neurosis and absent in those with psychosis, this is now regarded as too simplistic. Insight is now recognized to exist in a spectrum of varying degrees. David (1990) has considered insight to be composed of an awareness of one's own mental experiences, ability to recognize abnormal experiences as pathological, and compliance with treatment interventions. Insight is closely related to the neurological symptom of anosognosia. A patient who is suffering from a hemiplegia refuses to accept that he has lost the function of his limb. ('A'–absence, 'noso'–ill health or disease, 'gnosis'–awareness).

Sims A. *Symptom in the Mind*, 3rd edn. London: Elsevier Science, 2003, p. 206.
David AS. Insight and psychosis. *British Journal of Psychiatry* 1990; **156**: 798–808.

57. C. Depersonalization is the third most common symptom that is seen in patients attending psychiatric clinics. It is defined as a change in self awareness where the individual feels as if he is unreal. The 'as if' quality differentiates it from psychotic states. When a similar feeling occurs for objects and environment around an individual, it is termed as derealization (Mapother). It is always subjective, unpleasant, and invariably associated with affective change but preserved insight. Emotional numbing, loss of feelings of agency and self esteem, disturbed body image, altered perception of time, and disturbed sensory experiences of all modalities are reported.

Sims A. *Symptom in the Mind*, 3rd edn. London: Elsevier Science, 2003, p. 231.

58. D. The patient described here most probably suffers from depression with difficulty in expressing here feelings to others. Inability to verbally express emotional states (alexithymia) can partially explain symptoms of somatization occurring secondary to depression. In somatization disorder, recurrent, multiple, frequently changing somatic complaints are present for several years; this is not the case with the patient described in this question. Pathological changes in right cerebral hemisphere projections and failed thalamic feedback are also suggested but not proved as possible explanations for somatizing. It is suggested that the patients with first-rank symptoms of psychosis have difficulties in differentiating the 'source' of their experiences. They might misattribute internal mood state or self generated motor impulses to external sources, leading to a delusional elaboration.

Sims A. *Symptom in the Mind*, 3rd edn. London: Elsevier Science, 2003, p. 246.

59. C. Pathological gambling is defined as persistent, recurrent and problematic gambling behaviour associated with a preoccupation to gamble and spending increasing amounts of money in gambling. Patients often show a loss of control over gambling and pursue gambling at considerable expense of other activities of daily living. It is best regarded as an impulse control disorder together with kleptomania, intermittent explosive disorder and pyromania, etc. The gambling behaviour must not be directly due to manic episodes in order to be diagnosed as pathological gambling. It is not an overvalued idea; it is an abnormal behaviour and not merely an aberration of thought content. Pathological gambling is not an essential feature of antisocial personality.

DeCaria CM, *et al.* Diagnosis, neurobiology, and treatment of pathological gambling. *Journal of Clinical Psychiatry* 1996; **57** (Suppl. 8): 80–83.

60. E. Alexithymia is often accompanied by diminution of fantasy, reduced symbolic thinking, literal thinking concerned with details, difficulties in recognizing one's own feelings, difficulties in differentiating body sensations and emotional states, and complaints of robot-like existence. Amnesia is not a feature of alexithymia.

Sims A. *Symptom in the Mind*, 3rd edn. London: Elsevier Science, 2003, p. 309.

61. C. Out of body experiences, autoscopy, depersonalization, and transcendental experiences together in various proportions constitute a near death experience. The temporal–parietal junction may be the seat of pathological change in near death experience. The experience of seeing oneself from an external space is a feature of autoscopy. The detached, 'as if' quality of near death is linked to depersonalization.

Sims A. *Symptom in the Mind*, 3rd edn. London: Elsevier Science, 2003, p. 225.

62. B. In catatonic mutism comprehension is preserved and the patient may obey commands. It can range from full mutism to partial states where the patient mumbles and makes non-verbal vocalizations. Patients can move their vocalizing muscles – hence they can cough and clear their throats. Other catatonic signs are ambitendency (patient appears stuck in indecisive, hesitant movements), automatic obedience (exaggerated cooperation with examiner's request or incessant continuation of requested movement), and echopraxia/ echolalia (mimicking examiner's movements/ speech) etc.

Sims A. *Symptom in the Mind*, 3rd edn. London: Elsevier Science, 2003, p. 364.

63. D. Astasia–abasia refers to the inability to either stand or balance oneself. Patients exhibit a dramatic gait disturbance, inconsistent with focal neurological deficits. They can walk more or less normally though they cannot stand balanced. It is a dissociative conversion reaction similar to other pseudoneurological problems seen in conversion.

Sims A. *Symptom in the Mind*, 3rd edn. London: Elsevier Science, 2003, p. 252.

64. E. Hallucinations are not always pathological. Any normal person can experience hallucinations, for example hypnagogic hallucinations and hallucinations during bereavement. Even patients with very low IQ can experience these perceptual disturbances, as perception requires a lower-level cognitive processing. Even congenitally deaf patients can experience hallucinations, emphasizing the role of higher brain centres not lower sensory organs in producing the phenomenon.

Sims A. *Symptom in the Mind*, 3rd edn. London: Elsevier Science, 2003, p. 108.

65. E. An exaggeration of self-serving attribution bias is seen in psychosis. Patients excessively attribute hypothetical, positive events to internal causes (stable and global – grandiose) and hypothetical, negative events to external causes (stable and global – persecutory). When deluded patients were shown a sequence of black and white beads and were asked to decide which jar the sequence was probably drawn from (jar A had majority of black beads and B had majority of white), they came to a conclusion with far fewer beads in a given sequence than controls. They were also relatively overconfident about the accuracy of their judgement. This is hypothesized to be due to impaired probabilistic reasoning (the ability to generate hypothesis and test statistical probability). But later studies showed that when allowed to see as many beads as the controls, patients reached similar, correct conclusions – they were able to generate hypothesis and test the probability; the defect being deficient data gathering (less information before decision). This is called jumping-to-conclusion style of reasoning (JTC). Persecutory delusions reflect false beliefs about the intentions and behaviour of others that could arise from theory of mind deficits.

Sims A. *Symptom in the Mind*, 3rd edn. London: Elsevier Science, 2003, p. 130.
Also see
Blackwood NJ et al. Cognitive neuropsychiatric models of persecutory delusions. *American Journal of Psychiatry* 2001; **158**: 527–539.

66. A. Primary delusions do not carry any prognostic significance in schizophrenia, though they have diagnostic relevance. Primary delusions can occur in epileptic psychoses too. Primary delusional experiences occur more in acute stages of schizophrenia, and are rarely seen in chronic schizophrenia. In the chronic phase, original primary delusions are replaced largely by secondary delusions. The term secondary delusions refers to delusions that follow a primary delusion or follow other mental phenomena such as hallucinations, affective disturbances, etc.

Sims A. *Symptom in the Mind*, 3rd edn. London: Elsevier Science, 2003, p. 129.

...tive paramnesia is the delusional belief that a place or location has been ...existing in two or more places simultaneously, or that it has been 'relocated' to ...er site. It is one of the delusional misidentification syndromes and, although rare, is most commonly associated with acquired brain injury, particularly simultaneous damage to the right cerebral hemisphere and to both frontal lobes. It is also noted in patients with delirium.

David AS and Halligan PW. Cognitive neuropsychiatry: potential for progress. *Journal of Neuropsychiatry and Clinical Neuroscience* 2000; **12**: 506–510.

68. D. Among inpatients with schizophrenia, 25% have age disorientation. Age-disoriented patients are younger at first admission and have had a longer duration of stay than patients with a diagnosis of schizophrenia without age disorientation. Age disorientation may be a feature of a type of schizophrenic illness of early onset and poor prognosis.

Stevens M *et al*. Age disorientation in schizophrenia: a constant prevalence of 25 per cent in a chronic mental hospital population? *British Journal of Psychiatry* 1978; **133**: 130–136.

69. C. Bleuler argued that a cardinal feature of schizophrenic deterioration involved 'double registration' or 'double orientation'. According to him, in schizophrenic patients a delusional world exists where misinterpretations and threatening events are common. This is in addition to the existence of a 'real' world wherein life is near normal. These two orientations often get clearly separated in a long-standing, chronic schizophrenia patient.

Bleuler E. *Dementia Praecox or the Group of Schizophrenias*. New York: International Universities Press, 1950.

70. C. Akathisia is a subjective feeling of restlessness, with or without objective signs of restlessness. It can present with a sense of anxiety, inability to relax, jitteriness, pacing, rocking motions while sitting, and rapid alternation of sitting and standing. It can be measured using Barnes akathisia scale.

Sims A. *Symptom in the Mind*, 3rd edn. London: Elsevier Science, 2003, p. 368.

71. D. A gait disturbance seen in conversion disorder is called as astasia–abasia. It is a wildly ataxic, staggering gait accompanied by gross, irregular, jerky truncal movements, and thrashing and waving arm movements. Patients with the symptoms rarely experience a fall; even if they do, they do not get seriously injured. Posturing is maintaining an uncomfortable posture for a long time. Negativism is motiveless resistance to all movements; catatonia can also present itself as mitgehen – patient bends his limb even with a gentle finger push from the examiner like an 'angle poise lamp'. Ambitendence is tested by asking the patient to show his tongue – the patient will keep moving it in and out similar to a 'jack in the box'.

Sims A. *Symptom in the Mind*, 3rd edn. London: Elsevier Science, 2003, p. 365.

72. A. In neurological spasticity the tone is increased irrespective of passive or active movements. A patient with catatonia can use the affected limb or muscle group when needed with completely normal tone – for example running out when there is a fire. Negativistic phenomena, for example gegenhalten and mitgehen, are often distinguishing features of catatonia. Gegenhalten refers to the phenomenon where the patient resists movement of his or her extremities by the examiner. Mitgehen is said to be present when the patient moves in the direction of a slight push from the examiner in spite of the command to remain still. Catatonia persists in sleep and can continue for weeks without improvement. Catatonia is mostly seen in advanced primary mood or psychotic illnesses. Among inpatients with catatonic presentation, 25 to 50% are related to mood disorders and approximately 10% are associated with schizophrenia.

Sims A. *Symptom in the Mind*, 3rd edn. London: Elsevier Science, 2003, p. 365.

73. A. Some differences are reported in the quality of anhedonia experienced by patients who are depressed compared to patients with schizophrenia. In depression anhedonia is more physical – not able to enjoy listening to music, not able to enjoy going for walks, etc. In schizophrenia it is thought to be more social – that is not able to enjoy other's company, not feeling warm in personal relationships, etc. A longitudinal study by Blanchard *et al.* (2001) compared depressed patients and schizophrenia patients on a measure of social anhedonia; recovered depressed patients showed significantly less social anhedonia than schizophrenia patients on follow-up after 1 year. This suggests that anhedonia in depression is more of a state than a trait characteristic while it may be a trait characteristic in schizophrenia.

Joiner TE, *et al.* A test of the tripartite model's prediction of anhedonia's specificity to depression: Patients with major depression versus patients with schizophrenia. *Psychiatry Research* 2003; **119**: 243–250.
Blanchard JJ, Horan WP, Brown SA. Diagnostic differences in social anhedonia: a longitudinal study of schizophrenia and major depressive disorder. *Journal of Abnormal Psychology* 2001; **110**: 363–371.

74. C. Folie a deux is a shared delusion in which a psychotic person transfers his delusions to one or more people close to him. The non-psychotic 'victim' usually exhibits dependent traits on the primary patient. Separation of the pair can result in remission. The pair is usually a married couple or sisters/ brothers. Folie a deux can develop in any two persons with a close association with each other, irrespective of their actual relationship.

Sims A. *Symptom in the Mind*, 3rd edn. London: Elsevier Science, 2003, p. 140.

75. A. Obsessions by definition are ego dystonic – against ones values or ideals. Delusions often arrive as judgements or explanations, relieving a puzzled atmosphere that precedes them. In view of such 'relieving effect', delusions can be termed as ego syntonic. Overvalued ideas are adhered to and acted upon by the patient, making them ego syntonic.

Sims A. *Symptom in the Mind*, 3rd edn. London: Elsevier Science, 2003, pp. 337, 125.

76. B. Neologism refers to making up a totally new word that is not in a dictionary or using a known word with a completely different meaning. Perseveration refers to repetition of the same response to different stimuli. Perseveration also includes persistent repetition of specific words or concepts in the process of speaking. Such repeated responses may be meaningful but inappropriate, for example providing the same answer to different questions. Perseveration is seen as a frontal dysfunction. Verbigeration refers to meaningless and stereotyped repetition of words or phrases, as seen in schizophrenia. Verbigeration is also called cataphasia.

Sims A. *Symptom in the Mind*, 3rd edn. London: Elsevier Science, 2003, p. 181.

77. A. Both illusions and hallucinations are not necessarily pathological though they both are false perceptions, along with pseudohallucinations. Hypnagogic hallucinations are hallucinations occurring when going to sleep ('go' for 'go') these are usually auditory hallucinations. One's name being called by a familiar voice is the most common hypnagogic hallucination. This is also seen in narcolepsy–cataplexy where it can be visual or tactile too. Hypnopompic hallucinations (hallucinations when waking up) can occur in normal individuals. They also occur in glue sniffing, postinfective depression, children with febrile illness, and in phobic anxiety.

Sims A. *Symptom in the Mind*, 3rd edn. London: Elsevier Science, 2003, pp. 108, 112.

78. C. Wernicke's aphasia is also called jargon aphasia. Here the comprehension of a patient is limited but motor production is more or less preserved. This leads to error-prone language similar to the incoherence noted in schizophrenic speech disturbances. In Broca's aphasia the patient cannot produce fluent language although his comprehension is preserved. Alexia is inability to read words while agraphia is inability to write. Although schizophrenic speech disturbances can be deciphered from one's writing, this does not equate to having agraphia. Astereognosis refers to the inability to differentiate the character of an object by using a single perceptual modality, for example closing one's eyes and palpating a coin should be sufficient to discover the shape of the coin normally. This ability is absent in patients with astereognosis.

Covington MA *et al.* Schizophrenia and the structure of language: The linguist's view. *Schizophrenia Research* 2005; **77**: 85–98.

79. E. Paranoia is a loosely used term. Paranoia literally means 'beside the mind'. Paranoid delusions include any self-referential delusions such as referential delusions, persecutory delusions, grandiose delusions, hypochondriacal delusions, and nihilistic delusions. Some bizarre delusions are not self referential and are not classified as paranoid delusions, as in this question.

Sims A. *Symptom in the Mind*, 3rd edn. London: Elsevier Science, 2003, p. 144.

80. A. Catastrophic reaction is seen in demented patients who are asked to perform a task that is clearly beyond their cognitive capacity. They may become anxious, agitated, and angry. This is not a universal phenomenon. This occurs in some patients even if they do not have explicit awareness of their cognitive impairment.

Tiberti C *et al.* Prevalence and correlates of the catastrophic reaction in Alzheimer's disease. *Neurology* 1998; **50**: 546–548.

81. D. In this example, the best description for the patient's symptom of hearing voices is auditory hallucination. It cannot be somatic hallucination where touch sensations are involved. Abnormal bodily sensations called as 'cenesthesias' are well associated with psychopathological symptoms in schizophrenia. 'Cenesthopathic schizophrenia' is included but undefined within the category 'other schizophrenia' (F20.8) in the ICD-10 classification. Anosognosia refers to lack of awareness of having neurological deficits akin to loss of insight in schizophrenia. It is not somatization as this example describes a psychotic symptom. It is not extracampine as the patient's sensory field contains the source of the voice, that is his elbow is within the reach of his eyesight and auditory field.

Jenkins G and Röhricht F. From cenesthesias to cenesthopathic schizophrenia: a historical and phenomenological review. *Psychopathology* 2007; **40**: 5, 361.

82. B. Most psychopathological symptoms are noticeable in so-called normal population in the absence of diagnosable mental conditions. For example hypnagogic hallucinations are very common. Depersonalization can occur during fatigue in normal persons. Obsessions are noted in a child's developmental period even in the absence of any pathological processes. Amnesia is also common in the general population. But delusions are almost always pathological. It is argued that beliefs exist in a dimension from normalcy through overvalued ideas up to delusions. Even if this is true, when delusions are identified clinically, they almost always mean a pathological process.

Sims A. *Symptom in the Mind*, 3rd edn. London: Elsevier Science, 2003, p. 117–148.

83. A.   A parapraxis is an unintentional act that is explained in psychoanalytic terms as perfectly motivated but unconsciously determined failures of ego defence. According to Freud, parapraxes include failures of memory, slips of the tongue, mistaken identity or activities, etc. Confabulation refers to filling memory gaps in patients with organic memory difficulties such as Korsakoff's syndrome or dementia. A confabulating patient makes no attempt to correct the validity of his statement. In pseudologia fantastica, seen in Munchausen's syndrome and histrionic personality, 'fantastic' fluent lies are told without full awareness of their implications.

Berman D. Deliberate parapraxes. *International Review of Psycho-analysis* 1988; **15**: 381–384.

84. D.   In pronominal reversal a subject reverses the usage of the pronouns 'I' and 'you'. The patient may say 'You want a biscuit' when in fact she/ he wants a biscuit. This is seen in autistic children. This is more or less characteristic and not seen in other psychiatric illnesses as often as in autism. In conduction aphasia, repetition is affected while motor production of speech and comprehension are preserved. Pronominal reversal is not a part of schizophrenic speech disturbances or manic thought disorders.

Lee A. I, you, me, and autism: An experimental study. *Journal of Autism and Developmental Disorders* 1994; **24**: 155–176.

85. D.   Twirling is often noted in children with autism. The repetitive behaviours often seen in autism include hand flapping, finger flicking, rocking, jumping, and head banging. Repetitive use of a particular object or a part of the object is often observed in people at the lower functioning end of the autistic spectrum and in children rather than adults with autism. This is not a catatonic phenomenon.

Bodfish JW, *et al* Varieties of repetitive behaviour in autism; comparison to mental retardation. *Journal of Autism and Developmental Disorders* 2000; **30**: 237–243.

1. **Which of the following theories was NOT proposed by Sigmund Freud?**
   A. The topographical model of mind
   B. Affect trauma theory
   C. Individual psychology theory
   D. The structural model of the mind
   E. Psychosexual stages of development

2. **Which of the following is true about primary process thinking?**
   A. It fulfils the reality principle
   B. It fulfils the pleasure principle
   C. It is associated with delay in gratification
   D. It is ruled by rational thinking
   E. It is ruled by the concept of time

3. **All of the following are functions of ego EXCEPT**
   A. Accommodating the ego ideal
   B. Control and regulation of instinctual drives
   C. Rational judgement
   D. Mediation between the internal world and external reality
   E. Capacity to form mutually satisfying relationships

4. **Carol is undergoing psychotherapy. During her therapy sessions, she begins to argue with her therapist as she had argued with her deceased father. Which of the following phenomenon is she demonstrating?**
   A. Transference
   B. Resistance
   C. Free association
   D. Catharsis
   E. Repression

5. Which of the following refers to the mechanism by which several unconscious wishes can be combined into a single image in the manifest dream content?

A. Displacement
B. Symbolic representation
C. Secondary revision
D. Condensation
E. Dream work

6. According to Adler, a sense of inadequacy and weakness that is universal and inborn is called

A. Inferiority complex
B. Organ inferiority
C. Birth order theory
D. Masculine protest
E. Individual psychology

7. Which of the following is NOT a concept proposed by Melanie Klein?

A. Paranoid schizoid position
B. Reaction formation
C. Splitting
D. Depressive position
E. Projective identification

8. With which of the following developmental phases is Margaret Mahler associated?

A. Anal phase
B. Autistic phase
C. Conventional morality phase
D. Individuality vs inferiority phase
E. Operational stage

9. Avoiding the awareness of some painful aspect of reality by negating sensory data is called

A. Reaction formation
B. Projection
C. Denial
D. Suppression
E. Repression

10. Which of the following is NOT a mature defence mechanism?

A. Isolation
B. Altruism
C. Humour
D. Anticipation
E. Sublimation

11. **Which one of the following terms was coined by Mary Ainsworth?**

    A. Goodness of fit
    B. Anaclitic depression
    C. Transitional object
    D. Separation individuation
    E. Secure base

12. **Which of the following statements about attachment theory is INCORRECT?**

    A. Abused children do not develop attachments to their abusive parents.
    B. The attachment of the firstborn child is decreased by the birth of a second.
    C. Stranger anxiety develops by 8 months.
    D. Separation anxiety occurs by 10–18 months of age.
    E. Children brought up in extended families or with multiple caregivers are able to establish many attachments.

13. **A boy recognizes that the amount of water remains the same when transferred from a tall narrow glass to a wide-mouthed glass. Which stage of Piaget's developmental model is he likely to have attained?**

    A. Sensorimotor stage
    B. Preoperational stage
    C. Concrete operational stage
    D. Formal operational stage
    E. Conventional stage

14. **Which of the following is NOT a projective test?**

    A. Rorschach ink-blot test
    B. MMPI
    C. Sentence completion test
    D. Thematic apperception test
    E. Draw a person test

15. **A 30-year-old man presents to rehabilitation services following a head injury. Which of the following is the LEAST useful test to measure premorbid IQ in this patient?**

    A. Weschler's Adult Intelligence Scale
    B. National Adult Reading Test
    C. Cambridge Contextual Reading Test
    D. Spot the Word Test
    E. Wechsler Test of Adult Reading

16. **Choose a suitable test to assess frontal lobe functions in a man suffering from head injury:**
    A. Rey Osterreith test
    B. MMSE
    C. Wisconsin Card Sorting Test
    D. Stanford Binet Scale
    E. WAIS

17. **Among the WAIS subtests, performance on which of the following is relatively resistant to decline with ageing?**
    A. Digit symbol
    B. Digit span
    C. Block design
    D. Similarities
    E. Picture completion

18. **Which of the following is NOT a bedside cognitive test?**
    A. Halstead Reitan Battery
    B. Frontal Assessment Battery
    C. Verbal fluency
    D. Category test
    E. Go–no go test

19. **Which of the following scales used in antidepressant trials is most sensitive to detect any change in the severity of depression?**
    A. HAMD
    B. MADRS
    C. BPRS
    D. BDI
    E. PANSS

20. **While using a diagnostic rating scale, a psychologist tries to find the degree of correlation between one test item and the other items in the scale. What is he trying to measure?**
    A. Internal consistency
    B. Content validity
    C. Construct validity
    D. Split half reliability
    E. Test–retest reliability

21. The results of a child's IQ test relate significantly to the occupational success he achieves when he grows into an adult. The test is said to have a high

A. Construct validity
B. Predictive validity
C. Incremental validity
D. Face validity
E. Content validity

22. Which of the following is a structured diagnostic instrument used in population surveys to measure disease prevalence?

A. Young Mania Rating Scale
B. Positive and Negative Symptoms Scale
C. Hospital Anxiety and Depression Scale
D. Composite International Diagnostic Interview
E. Brief Psychiatric Rating Scale

23. Chris was confronted by a snake while hiking in a tropical forest. He later argued that the 'fear' he experienced was due to the tremors, muscle tension and sweating that occurred immediately upon seeing the snake. Which of the following theories is he using to explain the origin of his emotions?

A. Cannon–Bard theory
B. James–Lange theory
C. Two-factor theory
D. Opponent-process theory
E. Schachter–Singer theory

24. A psychiatrist wants to use a self-administered scale to assess the presence of depressive symptoms in a community-resident elderly patient. Which one of the following will he use?

A. The Centre for Epidemiologic Studies Depression Scale (CES-D)
B. The Carroll Rating Scale for Depression
C. The Geriatric Depression Scale (GDS)
D. Brief Psychiatric Rating Scale
E. Hamilton Depression Rating Scale

25. Matthew is a 3-year-old boy referred to the local Child and Adolescent Mental Health Services (CAMHS) team with a history of poor scholastic performance. Which of the following scales is considered appropriate to evaluate his intelligence quotient?

A. Stanford–Binet Scale
B. Denver Developmental Scale
C. Wechsler's WAIS-R
D. Wechsler's WISC III
E. Wechsler's WPPSI

26. **Classical conditioning has occurred when**

    A. Unconditioned stimulus produces unconditioned response
    B. Conditioned stimulus produces the conditioned response
    C. Unconditioned stimulus produces the conditioned response
    D. Conditioned stimulus produces another conditioned stimulus
    E. None of the above

27. **Repeated presentations of the conditioned stimulus in the absence of the unconditioned stimulus leads to a decrease in the strength of the conditioned response. This is known as**

    A. Extinction
    B. Generalization
    C. Higher order conditioning
    D. Inhibition
    E. Recovery

28. **When Little Albert was conditioned to be afraid of white rats he also came to fear white lab coats and other white objects. This phenomenon is known as**

    A. Extinction
    B. Satiation
    C. Generalization
    D. Discrimination
    E. Punishment

29. **The process by which the response to a stimulus declines with repeated exposure to that stimulus is known as**

    A. Conditioning
    B. Sensitization
    C. Boredom
    D. Generalization
    E. Habituation

30. **In a behavioural treatment, every time a person drinks alcohol, he is administered an electric shock. Which of the following principles underlie this treatment?**

    A. Cognitive therapy
    B. Punishment therapy
    C. Systematic desensitization
    D. Aversive conditioning
    E. Psychodynamic therapy

31. **A 19-year-old girl visits the London Dungeon. Her startle response increases with each fearful stimulus. This phenomenon is related to**

    A. Sensitization
    B. Habituation
    C. Systematic desensitization
    D. Relaxation
    E. Counter conditioning

32. **A 40-year-old lady is waiting to see her dentist after three painful extractions. She could hear the noise made by the dentist's drill. This makes her feel anxious. This anxiety could be termed as which one of the following?**

    A. Unconditioned stimulus
    B. Conditioned stimulus
    C. Conditioned response
    D. Unconditioned response
    E. None of the above

33. **Whenever Jack had to feed his pet dog, he would ring a bell in order to get its attention. He would stop ringing the bell before he served the meat. As days passed, the dog started salivating to the sound of the bell. Which of the classical conditioning paradigm is being used here?**

    A. Trace conditioning
    B. Backward conditioning
    C. Delayed conditioning
    D. Temporal conditioning
    E. Simultaneous conditioning

34. **Habitual consumption of paracetamol to relieve headache is related to which one of the following phenomena?**

    A. Aversion
    B. Positive reinforcement
    C. Classical conditioning
    D. Negative reinforcement
    E. Punishment

35. **Dave meets his girlfriend at a pub daily at 8 O'clock. As the time approaches, he keeps looking out for her more and more frequently through the window. This behaviour is suggestive of which of the following schedules of reinforcement?**

    A. Fixed interval
    B. Fixed ratio
    C. Differential
    D. Variable ratio
    E. Regular

36. **Which of the following schedules would most probably produce the greatest resistance to extinction?**

    A. Fixed interval
    B. Fixed ratio
    C. Variable ratio
    D. Differential ratio
    E. None of the above

37. **According to Skinner, a reinforcement is defined as any event that**

    A. Decreases a behaviour
    B. Increases a behaviour
    C. Increases or decreases a behaviour
    D. Is satisfying to the person
    E. Substitutes a punishment

38. **Which one of the following is a true statement about learned helplessness?**

    A. It was originally used as a cognitive model for depression.
    B. It occurs when met with uncontrollable aversive stimuli.
    C. It was first described by Beck.
    D. It is one of the cognitive triads of depression.
    E. None of the above.

39. **According to Seligman, people are more prone to develop phobia towards which one of the following?**

    A. Electric heaters
    B. Knives
    C. Hot ovens
    D. Electric iron
    E. Darkness

40. **A person who has never flown develops a fear of flying. Which one of the following best explains the above process?**

    A. Vicarious learning
    B. Flooding
    C. Operant conditioning
    D. Shaping
    E. Mowrer's hypothesis

41. **Which of the following is not a part of gestalt theory of perception?**

    A. Continuity
    B. Figure ground
    C. Proximity
    D. Shape constancy
    E. Closure

42. **Mark's neighbours were robbed when they were on holiday. On hearing the news, he said to his wife, "They are such a careless lot. They must have left their doors unlocked. This will never happen to us". He blamed the neighbours to minimize the apparent likelihood of a similar mishap to himself. This is best explained by**

    A. Defensive attribution
    B. Fundamental attribution error
    C. Actor–observer bias
    D. Stereotyping
    E. Self serving bias

43. **Dave attributed his success in the Part 1 exam to his hard work and extensive knowledge of the subject. But when he fails his Part 2 he blames it on the examination system being poorly standardized. This is an example of**

    A. The actor/observer effect
    B. Defensive attribution
    C. Stereotyping
    D. Self-serving bias
    E. Individualism

44. **Holiday makers who pay hundreds of pounds for a trip to a water theme park will rate the park favourably even if it was boring and mundane. This can be explained using which one of the following?**

    A. Self serving bias
    B. Learning theory
    C. Actor observer bias
    D. Dissonance theory
    E. Fundamental attribution theory

45. **A depressed person who failed his recent maths exam says 'I am stupid; I get everything wrong and will never pass any test'. The style of attribution in the above statement is**

    A. Internal, unstable, and specific
    B. Internal, stable, and global
    C. Internal, stable, and specific
    D. External, stable, and unspecific
    E. External, stable, and specific

46. **In a famous experiment of animal behaviour, newly hatched goslings were observed to follow the actively moving experimenter. This process, where some young animals learn to follow the first encountered moving object, is explained by which of the following?**

    A. Vicarious learning
    B. Learning theory
    C. Imprinting
    D. Cognitive dissonance theory
    E. Premack's principle

47. 'If you eat your spinach, you can have your dessert'. This is an example of which one of the following?

    A. Cognitive dissonance theory
    B. Attitude behaviour similarity theory
    C. Inoculation theory
    D. Attitude incongruity
    E. Premack's principle

48. Brian is dressed shabbily when he walks into the New Year party for junior doctors. When he finds everyone in the room to be dressed at their best, he feels depressed and unattractive. Which of the following can explain the above?

    A. Social inadequacy theory
    B. Ideas of self reference
    C. Social comparison effect
    D. Conformity theory
    E. Social incompetence effect

49. In a medical careers fair, most psychiatry trainees are noted to form a small social group on their own. The principle by which we categorize and identify ourselves as psychiatrists is explained by which one of the following?

    A. Social identity theory
    B. Self-reference effect
    C. Social comparison effect
    D. Social confirmity
    E. Social incompetence

50. Harry was recently diagnosed with an advanced carcinoma of the lung. He goes through a phase where he blames himself for the illness and asks 'why me?'. Which one of the following stages of reaction to impending death is he in?

    A. Denial
    B. Anger
    C. Bargaining
    D. Depression
    E. Acceptance

51. After breaking up with her boyfriend, Tanya says, "I don't think I have control over what is happening in my life". Which of the following statements would describe Tanya?

    A. She is a person with a high self esteem
    B. She is a person with a great sense of direction
    C. She is a person with an external locus of control
    D. She is a person with an internal locus of control
    E. She is a person who has achieved self actualisation

52. **A girl of age 2 years searches for her father when he leaves the room and is delighted when he enters the room. Which of the following phenomena explains this behaviour?**

   A. The girl has achieved object permanence
   B. The girl has achieved semiotic function
   C. The girl has achieved syllogistic reasoning
   D. The girl has achieved hypotheticodeductive reasoning
   E. The girl has achieved the principle of centration

53. **In Harlow's classical study of rhesus monkeys, the baby rhesus monkeys preferred soft-clothed, non-feeding surrogate mothers to hard, wire mesh, but food-providing surrogate mothers. This illustrated the concept of**

   A. Imprinting
   B. Individuation
   C. Insecure attachment
   D. Contact comfort
   E. Object relation

54. **Predictors of delinquency include which of the following?**

   A. Family history of aggression
   B. Family poverty
   C. Low IQ
   D. Lack of parental supervision
   E. All of the above

55. **Ryan is late for his WPBA meeting with his supervisor. After waiting for half an hour at the bus stop, he realizes that all buses in this route have been cancelled due to bad weather. He swears and kicks a can of Coke lying on the ground in anger. Which of the following would best explain this behaviour?**

   A. Ryan is angry with the litter on the ground
   B. Ryan is less polite when he is waiting for buses
   C. Frustration is associated with arousal
   D. Waiting for buses lead to an increase in blood pressure
   E. Bad weather leads to an increase in blood pressure

56. **Immigrant children in the UK tend to prefer the norms of their peers in the new culture compared to parental norms. Which one of the following could explain this?**

   A. Immigrant children don't like their original culture
   B. Immigrant children are compelled by their teachers to act like their peers
   C. Immigrant children want to pretend they are not immigrants
   D. Immigrant children need to act this way in order to survive at school
   E. Peers have more influence in transmitting cultural practices than parents

57. In spite of making a resolution to stop drinking, you place an order for a pint of lager when you see your friends place their order for drinks. Which of the following could explain the above phenomenon?

   A. Conformity
   B. Obedience
   C. Ignorance
   D. Acculturation
   E. Readiness

58. In a famous experiment conducted by Milgram in the 1960s, a 'teacher' was instructed by an 'experimenter' to deliver shocks of high voltage to the 'learner' every time he made a mistake. Which of these factors influenced the decision by the 'teacher' to obey the 'experimenter'?

   A. Diffusion of responsibility
   B. Perception of legitimate authority
   C. Persuasion techniques used by the authority
   D. Obedience to authority
   E. All of the above

59. There are five female PhD students living in a hostel for thirty at the university. Considering the girls to be the minority group, when will the group become influential in the hostel?

   A. If they are consistent with their views
   B. If they are joined by other girls and outnumber the majority
   C. When they complete their PhD
   D. When they spend a lot of money to influence the office bearers
   E. If the minority consist of older people

60. Tony was considered to be a silent, shy and well behaved boy by his family and friends. At a rock concert he attended on his own, Tony was thrown out because of disorderly behaviour, which they considered to be out of character. His behaviour can be explained by the theory that when we are in a group which guarantees anonymity, we tend to

   A. Accept our individuality
   B. Become frustrated
   C. Assume an alternate identity
   D. Become disinhibited secondary to deindividuation
   E. Hide from the rest of the group

61. A pianist is performing at a recital. According to the social facilitation theory which of the following is likely to happen?

   A. His performance can either improve or worsen in front of the audience
   B. His performance will improve when being observed
   C. His performance will worsen when being observed
   D. He will be supported by his community on contracting a disease
   E. He would be eligible for social benefits if he worked in a band rather than on his own

62. **A commercial sex worker receives an educational session regarding safe sexual practices from a health professional. She does not make any immediate change in her attitude or behaviour but agrees with the importance of such safe practice. Which of the following phases of Prochaska's Transtheoretical Model of Change is she in?**

    A. Preparation
    B. Precontemplation
    C. Contemplation
    D. Action
    E. Maintenance

63. **A frail-looking young man suddenly collapses on a busy market street and starts throwing a fit. In spite of the presence of many members of the public, no one comes forward to help him. Which of the following best explains the above observation?**

    A. Social equity norm
    B. Diffusion of responsibility
    C. Social exchange theory
    D. Guilt
    E. Altruism

64. **After receiving a small gift from a pharmaceutical representative, we feel indebted to prescribe the promoted drug. Which of the following could explain this behaviour?**

    A. Social exchange theory
    B. Equity and equality norm
    C. The reciprocal norm
    D. Social responsibility
    E. Guilt

65. **Margaret is 73-year-old. According to Erikson, she is most probably in the stage of**

    A. Integrity verses despair
    B. Intimacy verses isolation
    C. Trust versus distrust
    D. Autonomy verses shame and doubt
    E. Industry versus inferiority

66. Chris is planning his stag party. He knows the average number of cans of lager a person is likely to drink. From that he calculates the number of cans he will need to buy, and in turn the costs involved. During this complex mathematical calculation, he manipulates numbers in his memory. Which of the following types of memory is he most likely to be using?

    A. Iconic memory
    B. Implicit memory
    C. Episodic memory
    D. Working memory
    E. Semantic memory

67. A college student who last swam when he was 12 years old is surprised by his ability to swim when pushed into the pool during a party. Which of the following cognitive capacity could explain the above phenomenon?

    A. Procedural memory
    B. Retrospective memory
    C. State-dependent memory
    D. Eidetic memory
    E. Working memory

68. A student preparing for a physics test learned the definitions of the following terms an hour before the test in this order: Hubble's law, gravity wave, fusion, special relativity, string theory, and M theory. Which of the following definitions is he likely to forget?

    A. Fusion, special relativity
    B. Hubble's law and m theory
    C. String theory and m theory
    D. Hubble's law and gravity wave
    E. Gravity wave and string theory

69. The phase of human sexual response that occurs after desire is called

    A. Resolution phase
    B. Plateau phase
    C. Orgasmic phase
    D. Excitement phase
    E. Ejaculatory phase

70. According to Maslow's Hierarchy of Needs Theory, at the times of natural disasters which of the following will be the most appropriate intervention?

    A. Provision of food and shelter
    B. CBT to enhance self-esteem
    C. Group therapy to enhance love and belongingness
    D. Behavioural therapy to enhance safety behaviour
    E. Meditation to achieve self actualization

1. C. All of the theories listed in the question except Individual Psychology Theory were proposed by Sigmund Freud. Individual psychology theory was put forward by Alfred Adler. According to Freud's Affect Trauma Theory, feelings that are connected to unacceptable memories are strangulated by mental mechanisms leading to neurosis. Freud divided neurosis into 'actual' and 'psychoneurosis'. Actual neurosis manifested itself in anxiety neurosis or hypochondriasis. Psychoneurosis comprised of hysteria, obsessional neurosis, and phobias. Freud thought that psychoneurosis was amenable to psychoanalysis. In the Topographical Model, the mind is divided into the unconscious, preconscious, and conscious. The Structural Model of the Mind consists of the id, ego, and superego (a useful mnemonic is that S of structural model is shared with superego). Freud also came up with the stages of psychosexual development. In this, each stage of development is thought to build on and to subsume the accomplishments of the preceding stage: the oral stage (12 to 18 months of life), anal stage (18 to 36 months), phallic stage (3 to 5 years), latency stage (5 to 11 years), and genital stage (11 years to adulthood).

Sadock BJ and Sadock VA. *Kaplan & Sadock's Synopsis of Psychiatry: Behavioral Sciences/Clinical Psychiatry*, 10th edn. Lippincott Williams & Wilkins, 2007, p. 195–200.

2. B. Primary process thinking fulfils the pleasure principle. According to Freud, in the Topographical Model of the mind, the unconscious system is characterized by primary process thinking. Primary process thinking refers to a mode of thinking whose main aim is to facilitate wish fulfilment. It is governed by the pleasure principle and does not follow a logical course. The concept of time is not used to streamline primary process thinking. In addition, primary process thinking allows contradictions to exist simultaneously. The conscious system receives sense impressions from the outside world and follows secondary process thinking. This is ruled by time, rational–logical thinking, and the reality principle.

Sadock BJ and Sadock VA. *Kaplan & Sadock's Synopsis of Psychiatry: Behavioral Sciences/Clinical Psychiatry*, 10th edn. Lippincott Williams & Wilkins, 2007, p. 195.

3. A. The important functions of ego include the capacity to control the discharge of instinctual drives, the capacity to test reality, mediating between the id and the realities of the outside world (reality principle as against pleasure principle), and thus facilitating the formation of relationships. Judgement, which involves the ability to anticipate the consequences of actions, is also a function of the ego. In Freud's psychoanalytic theory of personality, the ego ideal is the part of the superego that includes the rules and standards for good behaviours (e.g. parental discipline).

Sadock BJ and Sadock VA. *Kaplan & Sadock's Synopsis of Psychiatry: Behavioral Sciences/Clinical Psychiatry*, 10th edn. Lippincott Williams & Wilkins, 2007, p. 200.

4. A.   This is an example of transference during psychotherapy. Transference is the process by which the patient displaces wishes and feelings toward persons from the past onto the analyst. Sometimes this leads to the emergence of resistance as patients experience the psychiatrist as a parental figure from the past (in this case the patient's dead father), and they seek to rebel against the perceived parental control. Resistance refers to an unconscious behaviour intended to frustrate the progress of therapy. Free association is the process where the client spontaneously expresses their thoughts and feelings as they occur. Repression is a defence mechanism.

Thambirajah MS. *Psychological Basis of Psychiatry*. Elsevier, 2005, p. 337.

5. D.   The phenomenon described is called condensation. According to Freud, a dream is the disguised fulfilment of an unconscious wish. Freud described two layers of dream content – the manifest and the latent. The manifest content is what the dreamer recalls; the latent content involves the unconscious thoughts and wishes that threaten to awaken the dreamer. The unconscious process by which latent dream content is changed into manifest dream is called the dream work. This dream work involves primary process revision (different from primary process thinking) and secondary revision/ elaboration. Primary process includes the mechanisms of condensation, displacement, and symbolic representation. Condensation, as described in this question, is the mechanism by which several unconscious wishes can be combined into a single image in the manifest dream content. Displacement refers to the transfer of energy from an original object to a different one. In symbolic representation of a wish or object, the original but highly unacceptable theme changes in physical qualities to a more acceptable object. This may be characterized by seemingly unrelated and absurd images. Secondary revision is the process by which dreams are made relevant and more rational when narrated to a third person.

Sadock BJ and Sadock VA. *Kaplan & Sadock's Synopsis of Psychiatry: Behavioral Sciences/ Clinical Psychiatry*, 10th edn. Lippincott Williams & Wilkins, 2007, p. 193

6. A.   Adler coined the term inferiority complex which is a sense of inadequacy and weakness that is universal and inborn. Masculine protest is the tendency to move from a passive, feminine role to a masculine, active role. A child's self esteem may be compromised by a physical defect; this phenomenon is called organ inferiority. According to Adler's birth order theory the firstborn child reacts with anger to the birth of siblings and struggles against giving up the powerful position of being the only child. The second-born child must always compete with the firstborn. This apparently results in lifelong influences on character and lifestyle. All the above terms, including individual psychology, were proposed by Alfred Adler.

Sadock BJ and Sadock VA. *Kaplan & Sadock's Synopsis of Psychiatry: Behavioral Sciences/Clinical Psychiatry*, 10th edn. Lippincott Williams & Wilkins, 2007, p. 214.

7. B.   Reaction formation is one of many Freudian defences. Kleinian defences can be remembered using the mnemonic (SIPDOG – splitting, introjection, projective identification, denial, omnipotence, and grandiosity). According to Klein, projection and introjection are the primary defence operations in the first few months of life. Soon after birth and thereafter, the infant experiences a fear that he is falling apart. This fear of fragmenting or disintegration is central to further Kleinian processes. To deal with this fear, the infant resorts to splitting, introjection, and projection. All events and perceptions are schemed into good and bad elements (splitting); the good part gets introjected, while bad part is projected onto the mother leading to persecutory anxiety. At this stage, the infant is in a paranoid–schizoid position, where the capacity to integrate varied experiences into unified concept is lacking. Soon the baby comes to know that the mother he loved (when feeding) and the mother he hated (when hurt) are one and the same. Now the infant becomes concerned that he might destroy the mother due to his aggressive impulses, and the infant is said to be in a grief-like depressive position. Projective identification is a Kleinian defence mechanism where unwanted feelings are projected to the other person, and he/she is made to feel and act accordingly.

Thambirajah MS. *Psychological Basis of Psychiatry*. Elsevier, 2005, p. 340.

8. B.   Margaret Mahler described the process by which children develop a separate identity from their mothers. She called this the theory of separation individuation (SI). Stages of separation individuation are: normal autism (birth to 2 months) where the infant sleeps most of the time, this phase is reminiscent of intrauterine life; Stage of symbiosis (2 to 5 months) where the mother and her child exist more or less as a single entity; differentiation (5 to 10 months), wherein physical and psychological distinctness from mother is gradually appreciated; practicing (10 to 18 months), where the child shows an increase in exploration of the outside world; rapprochement (18 to 24 months) where the child explores further away from the mother but on realizing the separation, comes back clinging; and object constancy (2 to 5 years) where the child realizes the permanence of the mother even when the mother is not from the vicinity (this is different from object permanence).

Sadock BJ and Sadock VA. *Kaplan & Sadock's Synopsis of Psychiatry: Behavioral Sciences/Clinical Psychiatry*, 10th edn. Lippincott Williams & Wilkins, 2007, p. 29.

9. C.   This is denial. The defence of denial is usually an unconscious process (I love that man becomes I do not love that man). Projection is where specific wishes, impulses, and aspects of self are imagined to be located in some other object external to oneself (e.g. a miser calling others 'misers'). Projection is thought to be involved in the formation of persecutory delusions. Repression is expelling or withholding an idea or feeling from consciousness. Primary repression is when the idea has never reached consciousness at all. Secondary repression is when it has reached the conscious level at some time in the past, but is now not available for conscious processing. Suppression is consciously or semiconsciously postponing attention and response to an impulse or conflict. This is a mature defence mechanism. Reaction formation is the transformation of an unacceptable impulse to the very opposite (I love that man becomes I hate that man).

Rycroft C. *A Critical Dictionary of Psychoanalysis*, 2nd edn. Penguin Reference, 2005, p. 125.
Sadock BJ and Sadock VA. *Kaplan & Sadock's Synopsis of Psychiatry: Behavioral Sciences/ Clinical Psychiatry*, 10th edn. Lippincott Williams & Wilkins, 2007, p. 207.

10. A. Isolation is a neurotic defence. It is separating an idea from the emotion that accompanies it. Defence mechanisms can be psychologically healthy or maladaptive, though their primary aim is to reduce a psychological conflict. Psychologically healthy mechanisms can be grouped as mature defences. Various mature defence mechanisms include sublimation, altruism, humour, suppression, and anticipation. Altruism is using constructive service to provide for others without any conscious direct or indirect benefits. Humour is the process of using comedy to express feelings and thoughts without personal discomfort. Anticipation is realistically planning for a predicted inner discomfort. For example, a man with a terminal illness prepares his advance directives. Sublimation is achieving gratification by altering a socially objectionable aim or objective to a socially acceptable one. For example training as a surgeon if you have a desire to cut and make others bleed!

Sadock BJ and Sadock VA. *Kaplan & Sadock's Synopsis of Psychiatry: Behavioral Sciences/Clinical Psychiatry*, 10th edn. Lippincott Williams & Wilkins, 2007, p. 207.

11. E. According to Mary Ainsworth, attachment in infants helps to reduce separation anxiety. Infants use the attachment figure as a 'secure base' around which they can explore the environment. Chess and Thomas proposed the theory of goodness of fit. They studied the innate psychological characteristics of every infant known as temperament. According to them, goodness of fit results when the expectations and demands from mothers match the temperamental characters of the infant. Margaret Mahler described the theory of separation individuation. Anaclitic depression (hospitalism) was first described by Rene Spitz in infants who had made normal attachments but were then suddenly separated from their mothers and placed in institutions or hospitals. These infants developed depression that was anaclitic (loss of dependent object) and recovered when their mothers returned. Sometimes, inanimate objects, called transitional objects (Winnicott) also serve as a secure base; these transitional objects are often soft toys or other commonly encountered things that often accompanies children as they investigate the world. For example, Hobbes in Calvin and Hobbes comic strips.

Thambirajah MS. *Psychological Basis of Psychiatry*. Elsevier, 2005, p. 280.

12. A. Abused children often maintain their attachments to abusive parents. Attachment behaviour can increase in the presence of hunger, sickness, or pain. Similarly when children are rejected by their parents or are afraid of them, their attachment may increase to some extent. Attachment develops in almost all children, but whether this is of a secure or insecure nature depends on multiple factors. Separation anxiety is a universal human developmental phenomenon emerging in infants less than 1 year of age and marking a child's awareness of a separation from his or her mother or primary carer. Separation anxiety peaks between 9 and 18 months and diminishes by about 2.5 years of age, enabling young children to develop a sense of comfort away from their parents in preschool.

Sadock BJ and Sadock VA. *Kaplan & Sadock's Synopsis of Psychiatry: Behavioral Sciences/Clinical Psychiatry*, 10th edn. Lippincott Williams & Wilkins, 2007, p. 137.

13. C. The concept of conservation develops in the stage of concrete operations. The primary sign that a child is still in the preoperational stage is that he or she has not achieved the concept of conservation or reversibility. Conservation is the ability to recognize that objects possess different compatible properties and the alteration of one property (e.g. height) does not necessarily alter other properties (e.g. volume). Conservation occurs in various dimensions – conservation of volume, quantity, number, area, and weight. Piaget's stages of cognitive development include sensorimotor stage, which begins at birth and lasts up to 2 years. Object permanence and insight is gained in this stage. During the stage of preoperational thought (2–7 years), the child develops symbolic play and semiotic function. Children in this stage are egocentric. In addition to conservation and reversibility, the child also develops syllogistic reasoning in the concrete operational stage (7–11 years). Formal operational stage (11 to thr end of adolescence), is characterized by the development of the capability of hypothetico-deductive reasoning.

Sadock BJ and Sadock VA. *Kaplan & Sadock's Synopsis of Psychiatry: Behavioral Sciences/Clinical Psychiatry*, 10th edn. Lippincott Williams & Wilkins, 2007, p. 136.

14. B. The projective tests of personality assessment make use of unstructured stimuli, for example inkblots or pictures from which stories have to be derived. It is thought that when confronted with a vague stimulus, subjects will introduce (project) some personality characteristics into the stimulus. This will be revealed not only in the way the ambiguity is perceived but also in the content of their responses. The Minnesota Multiphasic Personality Inventory (MMPI) is a self-report inventory with more than 500 true or false statements about oneself. It is an objective personality assessment instrument. The Rorschach Test is a standard set of ten inkblots which serves as the ambiguous stimulus for associations. In the Thematic Apperception Test (TAT) 20 stimulus cards depicting a number of scenes of varying ambiguity are used. Other projective tests include Draw a person test and sentence completion test.

Thambirajah MS. *Psychological Basis of Psychiatry*. Elsevier, 2005, pp. 195–196.

15. A. Wechsler Adult Intelligence Scale (WAIS) has a number of subtests, each tapping different aspects of intelligence. Verbal IQ is calculated based on the sum of the following subtests: vocabulary, similarities, arithmetic, digit span, information, and comprehension. Performance IQ is calculated from the sum of the following subtests: picture completion, digit symbol coding, block design, matrix reasoning, and picture arrangement. Three further subtests (symbol search, letter–number sequencing, and object assembly) have been added in later versions. National Adult Reading Test (NART), Cambridge Contextual Reading Test, Spot the Word Test, and Wechsler Test of Adult Reading are best used to test premorbid IQ. These measures are based on the observation that reading ability is relatively preserved in the face of organic cognitive impairment and is highly correlated with intellectual ability in the general population.

Johnstone EC *et al.*, eds. *Companion to Psychiatric Studies*, 7th edn. Churchill Livingstone, 2004, pp. 142–143.

16. C. The Wisconsin Card Sorting Test (WCST) is used to test set-shifting ability, which is thought to be a function of the frontal lobe. In Rey Osterreith Complex Figure Test (ROCFT) a complicated figure is presented and the subject is required to copy it. The original and copy are then removed and the subject is asked to draw the figure again from memory, after varying delay intervals. This is not specific for frontal lobe functions. Stanford Binet Scale measures general intelligence. Mini Mental State Examination (MMSE) is a test of general cognition. In fact, it does not include any specific tests for frontal lobe function.

Johnstone EC *et al.*, eds. *Companion to Psychiatric Studies*, 7th edn. Churchill Livingstone, 2004, p. 146.

17. E. Tests on WAIS are either 'hold' or 'no hold'. The so called 'hold tests' in WAIS are thought to reflect the use of old knowledge and are relatively resistant to the effects of brain damage and ageing. These include vocabulary, information, object assembly, and picture completion. 'No hold' tests require speed of response, working memory, or the creation of new relations between unrelated items. These are more likely to show early decline with ageing and cognitive impairment. These include digit symbol, digit span, similarities, and block design. This is the reason why WAIS is not the best test to measure premorbid intelligence.

Groth-Marnat G. *Handbook of Psychological Assessment*, 4th edn. John Wiley & Sons, 2003, p. 178.

18. A. The Halstead Reitan Battery is composed of seven to ten tests. The battery can differentiate those who are brain damaged from neurologically intact persons. It usually needs to be administered by a trained neuropsychologist and is time consuming. Frontal Assessment Battery is a battery of six tests used to test frontal lobe function at the bedside. It includes verbal fluency, similarities, Luria three-step test, go–no go tests, and a test of environmental autonomy. In category test the subject must discover the common theme in a set of pictures presented. Category test measures concept formation and abstract reasoning. It is one of the tests included in the Halstead Reitan Battery. Verbal fluency is measured using the FAS test.

Groth-Marnat G. *Handbook of Psychological Assessment*, 4th edn. John Wiley & Sons, 2003, p. 520.

19. B. The Hamilton Rating Scale for Depression (HAM-D) and the Montgomery-Åsberg Depression Rating Scale (MADRS) are two widely used depression scales. HAM-D is relatively limited in measures of sensitivity and multidimensionality but it is very popular. The MADRS (10 items), designed to be sensitive to treatment changes, is briefer and more uniform. A limitation of the MADRS is the lack of a structured interview, which may affect reliability. The HAM-D and the MADRS are often used conjointly as endpoints in depression trials. There are various versions of the HAM-D, ranging from 17 to 31 items. The Brief Psychiatric Rating Scale (BPRS) comprises 16 items rated from 0 (not present) to 6 (extremely severe) and includes symptoms such as somatic concern, anxiety, depressive mood, hostility, and hallucinations. The scale was developed essentially for psychosis but also includes symptoms of depression. Positive and Negative Symptoms Scale (PANSS) is not a scale to measure depressive symptoms. It is used to measure the severity of psychotic symptoms. The Beck Depression Inventory (BDI) is a 21 question, self-report inventory. It is not a very useful measure of change in severity of depression with treatment.

Iannuzzo R, Jaeger J, *et al*. Development and reliability of the HAM-D/MADRS Interview: An integrated depression symptom rating scale. *Psychiatry Research* 2006; **145**: 21–37.

20. A. Internal consistency is the degree to which one test item correlates with all other test items. Reliability is the consistency of a measuring instrument or the repeatability of a test. Inter-rater reliability is the likelihood that two raters will rate the same answer in the same way. Test–retest reliability is the degree to which a test will give the same result on two different occasions, separated in time. Parallel-form reliability is the extent to which two comparable versions of a test give the same result. Split-half reliability is when a test is notionally split in two and the two halves correlated with each other.

Gelder MG *et al*., eds. *New Oxford Textbook of Psychiatry*. Oxford University Press, 2000, p. 94.

21. B.   Validity is a property that refers to whether a test measures what it is supposed to measure. Predictive validity is the degree to which a test predicts some criterion that might be achieved in the future (e.g. whether a child's IQ test predicts occupational success when he/she grows into an adult). A test is said to possess good concurrent validity if scores on the test correlate with a gold standard or other diagnostic test used for the same purpose (e.g. if scores on HAMD are higher in those people with a severe rather than mild or moderate depressive disorder according to ICD 10, then HAMD is said to possess high concurrent validity). The above two types of validity together constitute criterion validity. Face validity refers to whether a test seems purposeful and sensible with regard to the tested domain to the person completing it. Content validity refers to the representativeness and relevance of the assessment instrument to the construct being measured. Construct validity checks whether a test measures a specified and well-defined construct. For example, if a test is measuring depression, there should not be clusters of items that seem to measure symptoms of mania; the test should correlate with other measures of depression (convergent validity); it should not correlate with measures that are irrelevant to depression (divergent validity).

Gelder MG et al., eds. New Oxford Textbook of Psychiatry. Oxford University Press, 2000, p. 94.

22. D.   The Young Mania Rating Scale (YMRS) comprises 11 items corresponding to the published core symptoms of mania. Four items are graded on a scale of 0–8 and have double weight; the remaining seven items are graded on a scale of 0–4. The Positive and Negative Symptom Scale (PANSS) is a 30-item rating instrument specifically designed to assess the psychopathology of schizophrenic patients. Subscores of the PANSS are positive, negative, general psychopathology, and affective symptoms composite scores. The Hospital Anxiety and Depression Scale (HADS) is a 14-item self-report scale that was developed originally to indicate the possible presence of anxiety and depressive states in medical outpatients. The Brief Psychiatric Rating Scale (BPRS) is a 16-item scale with nine general symptom items, five positive-symptom items, and two negative-symptom items. It is a clinician-completed scale often used in schizophrenia medication trials.

Spiegel R and Aebi HJ. Psychopharmacology: An introduction, 4th edn. Wiley, 2003, pp. 198–202.

23. B.   He is using the James–Lange theory of emotions. According to the James–Lange theory of emotion, the perception of the stimulus leads to physiological arousal. The interpretation of the physiological arousal leads to the affective experience of the emotion. For example, 'I feel afraid because my heart is pounding'. According to Cannon–Bard theory, perception of an emotionally relevant stimulus leads to the physiological and emotional arousal at the same time. Cannon and Bard attributed this to stimulation of the hypothalamus and the autonomic areas at the same time. In the Schacter–Singer theory (two factor theory), a person labels the pounding of the heart as fear because he appraises the situation of being in the midst of a snake as dangerous. So according to Schacter, the same physiological feeling can elicit different emotions depending upon the appraisal made by the subject from his situation. For example, pounding of the heart can be due to fear of the snake, anxiety secondary to exams and joy (or fear!) of meeting one's spouse. Opponent-process theory is a theory of colour vision.

Sadock BJ and Sadock VA. Kaplan & Sadock's Synopsis of Psychiatry: Behavioral Sciences/ Clinical Psychiatry, 10th edn. Lippincott Williams & Wilkins, 2007, p. 190.

24.A. The CES-D is the most widely used screening instrument for depression in community-resident elderly because of the availability of normative population data. The GDS (Geriatric depression scale), developed specifically to screen older persons for the presence of depressive symptoms, has not been standardized for use in community populations. The Carroll Rating Scale for Depression, based on the Hamilton Depression Scale, has not been used extensively in elderly people. HAM-D includes many somatic elements of depression, which are often positive even in the absence of depression among elderly people due to high prevalence of physical health problems. It is observer rated and not self administered. BPRS does not look for the presence or absence of depression.

Radloff LS. The CES-D scale: A self report depression scale for research in the general population. *Applied Psychological Measurement* 1977; **1**: 385–401.

25.A. The Stanford–Binet scale is suitable for children between 2 and 4 years since it does not rely exclusively on language. It is also applicable for other age groups. The Denver Developmental Scale is used to assess the attainment of developmental milestones in children up to age 5. The WAIS-R (Wechsler Adult Intelligence Scale) is used for individuals aged 17 and over. The WISC III (Wechsler Intelligence Scale for Children) is useful for evaluating children aged 6–16. The WPPSI (Wechsler Preschool and Primary Scale of Intelligence) is used for children aged 4–6.

Groth-Marnat G. *Handbook of Psychological Assessment,* 4th edn. John Wiley & Sons, 2003, pp. 132–133.

26.B. The unconditioned stimulus (UCS) is a stimulus that evokes an unconditioned response (UCR) without previous conditioning, for example in the classic Pavlov's paradigm, salivation (UCR) with food (UCS). UCR is not a learned response. Conditioned stimulus (CS) is a previously neutral stimulus that has acquired the capacity to evoke a conditioned response (CR) , for example the bell is the CS that is paired with food (UCS) which later elicits the salivation (now a CR). A first CS (CS1) that has previously been paired with a UCS can support conditioning to a second CS (CS2) when the CS2 and CS1 are paired together. Thus CS2, never directly paired with the UCS, still elicits a CR. This is higher-order conditioning.

Thambirajah MS. *Psychological Basis of Psychiatry*. Elsevier, 2005, p. 8.

27.A. Extinction is the process by which CR is eliminated. After conditioning a CS to elicit a CR, repeated, subsequent delivery of the CS without the UCS extinguishes the CR. Three factors influence the extinction of the CR. In general, the stronger the CS–CR bond, the slower the extinction of the CR. When the CS is only occasionally presented during initial conditioning, resistance to extinction is increased. As the duration of the CS exposure in extinction increases, the CR weakens proportionately. Spontaneous recovery is the reappearance of an extinguished response after a period of non-exposure to the conditioned stimulus.

Weiten W. *Themes and Variations*, 3rd edn. Brooks/Cole, 1995, p. 218.

28. C. Stimulus generalization occurs when an organism that has learned a response to a specific stimulus responds in the same way to new stimuli that are similar to the original stimulus. In this case, the colour white serves as the similarity between rats and lab coats. The closer the new stimuli are to the original conditioning stimulus, the greater the likelihood of generalization. Stimulus discrimination occurs when an organism that has learned a response to a specific stimulus does not respond in the same way to new stimuli that are similar the original stimulus. For example, a dog which wags its tails when it hears your car approaching the porch may initially wag when any car passes by (generalization). But as time goes, your faithful dog learns to discriminate the distinct sound of your car from your father-in-law's car, who you may not like very much! The 'Little Albert' experiment mentioned in this question was conducted by Watson and Rayner in 1920. Albert was 11 months and 3 days old at the time of the first test. Because of his young age, the experiment today would be considered unethical.

Johnstone EC et al., eds. *Companion to Psychiatric Studies*, 7th edn. Churchill Livingstone, 2004, p. 107.
Harris B. Whatever happened to Little Albert? *American Psychologist* 1979; **34**: 151–160.

29. E. Habituation and sensitization are two fundamental learning processes. In each case, animals change their reactions to a stimulus with repeated stimulation. Habituation is defined as a decrease in responsiveness to a stimulus, for example you may get habituated to the pressure on your toes from a new shoe when you wear it regularly. Sensitization refers to an increase in reactivity to the stimulus on repeated exposure, for example repeated listening to the new ring tone of your mobile may make you attend to the call quicker than on the first few days of buying the phone.

Johnstone EC et al., eds. *Companion to Psychiatric Studies*, 7th edn. Churchill Livingstone, 2004, p. 107.

30. D. Aversive conditioning makes use of the classical conditioning paradigm. Here an unwanted behaviour is paired with an aversive stimulus, thus eliciting an aversive response. Here the shock is not given as a punishment but it is given as an unconditioned stimulus (UCS) to which an unconditioned response (UCR), pain, will be elicited. By repeated pairing of alcohol (conditioned stimulus, CS) with electric shock, the pain (aversion) becomes a conditioned response (CR). Later drinking alcohol (CS) alone is expected to produce the CR of aversion and pain. Typically, a short, delayed conditioning paradigm is used (see Question 33), that is the patient is asked to pour alcohol into his mouth and half a second later a shock is delivered to his hand via an electrode.

Thambirajah MS. *Psychological Basis of Psychiatry*. Elsevier, 2005, pp. 10–11.

31. A. This is an example of sensitization. Systematic desensitization is a therapy based on conditioning procedures that can be effective in the elimination of conditioned fear and the reduction of phobic behaviour. It has three steps: relaxation training, hierarchy formation, and exposure to the stimuli. By remaining relaxed while imagining the lowest item in the hierarchy, the fear of that situation or object is counter conditioned. In a similar fashion counter conditioning then proceeds to situations higher in the hierarchy.

Johnstone EC et al., eds. *Companion to Psychiatric Studies*, 7th edn. Churchill Livingstone, 2004, p. 107.

32. C. The anxiety produced by the sound is the conditioned response (CR). Pain produced by the situation of drilling is the UCR. This is called fear conditioning and is one of the theories to account for the origin of phobias. When this classical conditioning paradigm is combined with operant conditioning, in the form of avoidance (negative reinforcement), a phobia is likely to have developed. So in fully developed dental phobics, not only there is anxiety produced by the noise of the drill, but also avoidance of the situation by not keeping the appointment (or waiting outside the waiting room). The stimulus itself may become generalized to a fear of all drills.

Thambirajah MS. *Psychological Basis of Psychiatry*. Elsevier, 2005, pp. 15–16.

33. A. This is an example of trace conditioning. There are five paradigms that are used in classical conditioning. They differ with respect to how a CS is paired with a UCS. In delayed conditioning, the onset of the CS precedes the onset of the UCS and termination of the CS occurs either with the onset of the UCS or during UCS presentation. In trace conditioning, the CS is presented and terminated prior to the onset of the UCS. In simultaneous conditioning, the CS and the UCS have onsets at the same time. In backward conditioning, the UCS is presented and terminated before the onset of the CS. In temporal conditioning, the UCS is presented at regular time intervals allowing the timing of the UCS to serve as the CS eliciting the CR. Short delayed conditioning is the best arrangement that facilitates the acquisition of most conditioned responses. Ideally the delay between the onset of CS and UCS should be about half a second.

Weiten W. *Themes and Variations*, 3rd edn. Brooks/Cole, 1995, p. 218.
Thambirajah MS. *Psychological Basis of Psychiatry*. Elsevier, 2005, pp. 3, 4.

34. D. Negative reinforcement occurs when a response is strengthened because it is followed by the removal of an aversive stimulus. In this case, the headache. Other types of negative reinforcement include escape and avoidance learning. The term negative reinforcement should not be confused with punishment, which is an event following a behaviour which reduces the behaviour, for example stopping rash driving after getting a speeding ticket. Positive reinforcement occurs when a response is strengthened because it is followed by the presentation of a rewarding stimulus. For example a prize given for a desired behaviour increases the behaviour. It should be noted that both positive and negative reinforcements increase the behaviour in question. Punishment, on the other hand, decreases the behaviour.

Weiten W. *Themes and Variations*, 3rd edn. Brooks/Cole, 1995, p. 230.

35. A. In operant conditioning, the relationship between a response and the likelihood of reinforcement is known as a schedule of reinforcement. There are two major classes of schedules: (1) ratio schedules require a certain number of responses to produce reinforcement, and (2) interval schedules require a certain amount of time to elapse since the last reinforced response. Both types are subdivided into fixed and variable. In a fixed ratio schedule, a fixed number of responses produce the reinforcement. For example, a rat is reinforced every 10 times it presses the lever. In variable ratio schedule, an average number of responses produce the reinforcement. It is similar to fixed, but here the frequency of behaviour required to elicit the reinforcement changes after each reinforcement, for example slot machine in the casino pays off once every 10 times on an average, so it can take five attempts for some while 15 attempts for others. The fixed interval schedule involves a contingency in which reinforcement for a response is produced only after a specified period of time has elapsed since the previous reinforced response, for example students earn grades after a test every 3 weeks. In this case, they don't read during the initial weeks, but start reading just before the exam, that is the response increases just before the reinforcement. The variable interval schedule is the same as a fixed interval schedule, except that the interval changes after each reinforced response, for example repeatedly dialling a phone number till one gets through to a lucky draw contest. When reinforcement depends on both time and number of responses, the contingency is called a differential reinforcement schedule.

Thambirajah MS. *Psychological Basis of Psychiatry*. Elsevier, 2005, p. 14.

36. C.　Reinforcement for an operation in operant conditioning can be provided at various schedules. When every operation is reinforced this is called continuous schedule. Intermittent reinforcement can occur at a fixed ratio (every third operation is rewarded), variable ratio (random rewards for operations), fixed interval (operation that takes place at every fourth minute is rewarded), or variable interval (random time intervals for reward delivery). Though learning is relatively slower, resistance to extinction increases with partial reinforcement. The variable ratio schedule is the most difficult to extinguish. This is the principle behind slot machines and gambling addiction.

Thambirajah MS. *Psychological Basis of Psychiatry*. Elsevier, 2005, p. 14.

37. B.　Reinforcement occurs when an event following a response increases an organism's tendency to make that response. Primary reinforcers are events that are inherently reinforcing because they satisfy biological needs, for example food, water, sex, etc. Secondary or conditioned reinforcers are events that acquire reinforcing qualities by associating with primary reinforcers, for example money, good grades in exams, praise, etc.

Weiten W. *Themes and Variations*, 3rd edn. Brooks/Cole, 1995, p. 222.

38. B.　The concept of learned helplessness was proposed by Martin Seligman. Seligman noted that when an animal is confronted with aversive stimuli from which escape is impossible, the animal stopped trying to escape. This was initially used as a behavioural model for depression. Cognitive triad of depression was first proposed by Aaron T Beck. The triad consists of a negative view of self, the world, and the future, that is worthlessness, helplessness, and hopelessness. The triad forms the theoretical basis for cognitive therapy in depression.

Gross R. *Psychology: The Science of Mind and Behaviour*, 5th edn. Hodder Arnold, 2005, p. 790.
Thambirajah MS. *Psychological Basis of Psychiatry*. Elsevier, 2005, p. 16.

39. E.　Seligman's concept of stimulus preparedness involves a species-specific inclination to be conditioned in certain ways. He believed that this was a product of evolution and was necessary for the survival of species. Accordingly, genuine threats to the survival of our ancestors easily elicit phobic responses in humans, for example snakes, darkness, etc. Hence it is more common for people to develop snake phobias than to develop sheep phobias, even though they may never have had any direct adventure with a snake.

Johnstone EC *et al.*, eds. *Companion to Psychiatric Studies*, 7th edn. Churchill Livingstone, 2004, p. 107.

40. A.　Observational or vicarious learning (proposed by Albert Bandura) occurs when one's behaviour is influenced by observing models. A model may be any significant person or even an incident on television. So a person may develop a fear of flying after seeing an air disaster in a movie or a hijacking event on the television. Shaping is the progressive reinforcement of responses that are close to a desired response. This progressive reinforcement is continued until the desired response (usually a complex behaviour) is elicited. It is based on operant conditioning and works as the principle behind training animals to do circus tricks. Mowrer's hypothesis puts forth a two-staged acquisition process for phobia wherein, initially, classical conditioning associates a fear response to a neutral stimulus. Later, through operant conditioning, this fear is maintained, as avoidance of the feared stimulus serves as a potential negative reinforcer. Note that in the scenario portrayed in this question there has been no previous exposure to the feared stimulus (flying). Hence operant conditioning and Mowrer's hypothesis can be safely ruled out.

Johnstone EC *et al.*, eds. *Companion to Psychiatric Studies*, 7th edn. Churchill Livingstone, 2004, p. 108.

41. D. Gestalt principle of perception is a theory of sensory information processing. Initially, any figure must be separated from its background. This is called the figure ground principle. The actual perception of the figure as a whole usually follows the principles of grouping. These are proximity, similarity, continuity, simplicity, common fate, and closure. The gestalt principle is based on the top-down processing of perception, that is a whole picture makes more sense and is easier to understand than parts of the same picture. In a similar sense, presenting letters one by one in random order of R, O, K, W, is more difficult to process than presenting the word WORK. The opposite, bottom-up processing, refers to a progression from individual elements to the whole. For example, bottom-up processing occurs when children initially learn to spell words. They initially identify each letter and then go on to learn to the whole word. A perceptual constancy is the tendency to experience an object as the same thing in spite of continually changing sensory input, for example we recognize an open door and a closed door as a door, irrespective of the differing geometry. Perceptual constancy includes concepts of size constancy, shape constancy, etc.

Gross R. *Psychology: The Science of Mind and Behaviour*, 5th edn. Hodder Arnold, 2005, p. 244.

42. A. Defensive attribution is a tendency to blame victims for their misfortune, so that one feels less likely to be victimized in a similar way. It also helps people to maintain their belief that they live in a just world. For example assuming that victims of a burglary were careless. Attributions are inferences that people draw about causes of events and behaviours – both their own and other person's behaviours. Internal attribution attributes the cause to personal disposition. External attributions ascribe the cause to situational demands and environmental reasons. Fundamental attribution error refers to the process where an observer attributes others' negative behaviour to their internal attributes. The systematic bias in attribution, when one's own behaviour is assessed favourably compared to others' behaviours, is called the actor–observer bias.

Thambirajah MS. *Psychological Basis of Psychiatry*. Elsevier, 2005, p. 218.

43. D. Self-serving bias is said to occur when a person attributes his success to personal factors, while attributing his failures to external factors. It is a type of fundamental attribution error. Illusory correlation occurs when people estimate that they have encountered more confirmations of an association than they have actually seen, for example after meeting one dishonest lawyer, a person makes a statement 'I have never seen an honest lawyer'. Stereotypes are widely held beliefs that people have certain characteristics because of their membership in certain groups, for example lawyers are dishonest. Individualism is the process of defining one's identity in terms of personal attributes rather than group membership. Collectivism is when one's identity is defined in terms of group membership. Fundamental attribution error is seen less in collectivist cultures. Self-serving bias is seen more in individualistic Western culture. Naïve psychology, or common sense psychology, refers to certain propositional beliefs we hold about the actions and intentions of others in every-day life. These beliefs are socially conditioned and are necessary for human interaction. For example when someone waits in a queue to buy a train ticket, we infer that the person is travelling somewhere. These propositional ascriptions are not experimentally tested but heuristic and, in some cases, probabilistic assumptions.

Thambirajah MS. *Psychological Basis of Psychiatry*. Elsevier, 2005, p. 218.
Gross R. *Psychology: The Science of Mind and Behaviour*, 5th edn. Hodder Arnold, 2005, p. 402.

44. D. This is an example of postdecisional cognitive dissonance. Cognitive dissonance occurs when there is discord among a person's different beliefs or behaviours. When a person experiences cognitive dissonance he/she changes his/her thinking or behaviour to lessen the disharmony. For example the owner of an expensive Porsche experiences a cognitive dissonance when the car breaks down on the motorway. He always believed that 'Porsches do not break down'. Now he looks for alternative explanations. As a result of this dissonance he may change his belief as follows: 'This is just a one-off event; this cannot happen again'.

Thambirajah MS. *Psychological Basis of Psychiatry*. Elsevier, 2005, pp. 222–224.

45. B. According to Seligman's modified theory of learned helplessness, depressed patients usually have attribution styles that are internal, stable, and global. It is 'internal' as they make causal attributions to internal personal traits rather than external events. These attributions are called stable as they are fixed and held in spite of evidence to the contrary. They are global as they encompass all areas of functioning, for example in the scenario in Question 45, the person attributes to himself being stupid (negative and internal), will never pass a test (stable), and gets everything wrong (global).

Thambirajah MS. *Psychological Basis of Psychiatry*. Elsevier, 2005, p. 219.

46. C. Imprinting, first described by Konrad Lorenz is a form of learning that occurs in the very early life of certain animals. The exposure to a stimulus must occur during a critical period, though this could be of a short duration. Imprinted associations are very resistant to change. Lorenz described newly hatched goslings that are programmed to follow a moving object, typically the mother, but in this experiment followed Lorenz because he was the first moving object they came in contact with. Imprinting does not depend on any reinforcement and it is not clear whether this occurs in human infants and all primates.

Sadock BJ and Sadock VA. *Kaplan & Sadock's Synopsis of Psychiatry: Behavioral Sciences/Clinical Psychiatry*, 10th edn. Lippincott Williams & Wilkins, 2007, p. 159.

47. E. Premack's principle is based on the concept that high-frequency behaviour can be used to reinforce a low-frequency behaviour. In this particular example, children eat a lot of sweets (high-frequency behaviour), but this can be made contingent on eating their greens (low-frequency behaviour), thus increasing this behaviour (also called the Grandma's rule).

Sadock BJ and Sadock VA. *Kaplan & Sadock's Synopsis of Psychiatry: Behavioral Sciences/Clinical Psychiatry*, 10th edn. Lippincott Williams & Wilkins, 2007, p. 146.

48. C. The Social Comparison Theory was developed by Festinger. It refers to an individual's drive to look around him in the society to evaluate his own abilities. When the individual compares himself to someone who is deemed socially better, it is called an upward social comparison. The opposite is called a downward social comparison. Often individuals try to compare themselves with someone with whom they should be reasonably similar, for example their peers. The Self-Referential Encoding (SRE) effect holds that information relating to the self is preferentially encoded and organized above other types of information.

Gross R. *Psychology: The Science of Mind and Behaviour*, 5th edn. Hodder Arnold, 2005, pp. 469, 433.

49. A. Social Identity Theory is concerned with explaining when and why individuals act as part of social groups. At the psychological level it tries to answer why individuals identify with the group that they are a part of. At a social level, it tries to explain why individual interactions are different from interaction between individuals as members of different groups. The main concepts of social identity include:

1. Categorization, where we categorize ourselves, for example 'Doctors can be physicians or surgeons' (this categorization allows significant assumptions to be drawn about one's identity);
2. Identification, where we associate with our specific group (in-groups), which serve to raise our self esteem, for example 'I am a surgeon and not a physician';
3. Comparison, where we compare our groups with other groups, usually with a bias favouring ourselves, for example 'Psychiatrists are better thinkers than surgeons'.

Social comparison refers to comparing oneself with one's peers while social coherence refers to identifying commonalities with the wider social network.

Gross R. *Psychology: The Science of Mind and Behaviour*, 5th edn. Hodder Arnold, 2005, p. 433.

50. B. The stage of dying described in this scenario corresponds to that of 'anger'. Kubler-Ross described the five stages of dying in her book 'Death and dying'. According to her theory, people's reaction to impending death follows five stages. The first one being a state of denial, where the person is in a state of shock and denies the diagnosis of terminal illness. He may blame the doctor for giving him a wrong diagnosis. The second stage is that of anger, where the person becomes irritable and frustrated, often asking the question 'Why me? ' blaming himself or even God for being in the state he is in. In the third stage of bargaining, the person may try to negotiate with the doctor or family members or God to alleviate his illness in exchange of good deeds. Stage four is that of depression, where the cognitive triad of hopelessness, helplessness, and worthlessness are demonstrable. This may require treatment with antidepressant if severe. The fifth and final stage is of acceptance where the patient acknowledges and comes to terms with the inevitability of his/ her death.

Sadock BJ and Sadock VA. *Kaplan & Sadock's Synopsis of Psychiatry: Behavioral Sciences/Clinical Psychiatry*, 10th edn. Lippincott Williams & Wilkins, 2007, p. 62.
Kubler-Ross E. *On Death and Dying*. New York: Macmillian, 1969.

51. C. Locus of control is a concept proposed by Julian Rotter as a part of his social learning theory of personality. Those with external locus of control attribute their successes and failures to external factors, for example luck, fate, etc. They believe that outcomes are largely out of their control. Those with an internal locus of control believe that success and failures are determined by their own action and abilities. There is some evidence suggesting that people with a high external locus are prone to more psychological problems. People with a high internal locus of control tend to be more successful. People with an external locus of control may be more prone to develop an equivalent of learned helplessness. For a given subject, locus of control may differ based on the issue considered. Consider the example – a person may feel that the political situation in his country is uncontrollable (external), but his own personal situation may be considered to be well under his control (internal).

Gross R. *Psychology: The Science of Mind and Behaviour*, 5th edn. Hodder Arnold, 2005, p. 203.

52. A. Object permanence is the understanding that an object tends to exist even when it cannot be seen or touched. Piaget argued that very young infants did not have a concept of durability of objects, that is 'out of sight is out of mind'. He claimed that the concept of object permanence was achieved by infants only during the late sensorimotor stage (at around 9 months). More recently this has been challenged by some studies (Hood and Willatts), which state that infants may start developing object permanence even as early as 5 months. Semiotic function is the process where children start to use a symbol or sign to represent an object. For example drawing is a semiotic function which may signify something in the real world. Semiotic function emerges during the preoperational stage. Syllogistic reasoning is the process by which a logical conclusion is formed from two ideas. For example crows are birds (premise 1); birds lay eggs (premise 2); therefore crows lay eggs (conclusion). This is developed during the stage of concrete operations. Centration is the tendency to focus on just one aspect of a problem, neglecting other important features. Centration is considered to be one of the basic flaws in cognition, which leads to the inability of the child to understand the concept of conservation in preoperational stage. Hypotheticodeductive reasoning is considered to be the highest order of reasoning, where a person can develop a hypothesis and test it to reach conclusions. This function usually develops in the formal operational stage according to Piaget.

Sadock BJ and Sadock VA. *Kaplan & Sadock's Synopsis of Psychiatry: Behavioral Sciences/Clinical Psychiatry*, 10th edn. Lippincott Williams & Wilkins, 2007, pp. 135–137.

Hood B and Willatts P. Reaching in the dark to an object's remembered position: Evidence for object permanence in 5-month-old infants. *British Journal of Developmental Psychology* 1986; **4**: 57–65.

53. D. Harry Harlow in his famous experiments in the 1950s separated rhesus monkeys from their mothers during their first weeks of life. Harlow substituted a surrogate mother made from wire or cloth for the real mother. The infants preferred the cloth-covered surrogate mother, which provided contact comfort, to the wire-covered surrogate, which provided food but no contact comfort. Harlow suggested that the infant monkeys depended on its mother not only for nourishment, but also for physical warmth and emotional security, which he termed 'contact comfort'. This is an important concept in attachment. Harlow's experiment refuted the hypothesis that attachment occurs as a result of positive reinforcement to feeding. Imprinting is associated with Konrad Lorenz and geese. Harlow was not an object relation theorist; Klein, Fairburn, and Guntrip are considered to be object relation analysts.

Sadock BJ and Sadock VA. *Kaplan & Sadock's Synopsis of Psychiatry: Behavioral Sciences/Clinical Psychiatry*, 10th edn. Lippincott Williams & Wilkins, 2007, p. 28.

54. E. Farrington *et al.* (see reference below) in their Cambridge study in delinquent behaviour identified the following predictors of delinquency:

1. Antisocial behaviour and conduct traits beginning in early childhood (before age of 8);
2. Inattention (symptoms suggestive of ADHD);
3. Low intelligence and poor school attainment;
4. Family criminality;
5. Family poverty;
6. Large family size; and
7. Harsh parenting style with lack of parental supervision.

Farrington DP. Key results from the first forty years of the Cambridge Study in Delinquent Development. In: TP Thornberry and MD Krohn, eds. *Taking Stock of Delinquency: An Overview of Findings from Contemporary Longitudinal Studies*. New York: Kluwer Academic/ Plenum Press, 2002, 137–183.

55. C. John Dollard's frustration–aggression hypothesis states that aggression invariably stems from frustration and frustration in turn leads to aggression by arousing an individual. But frustrated individuals may react in various ways including resignation, depression, and despair. As a corollary not all aggression results from frustration, for example aggression exhibited during sporting activities such as boxing.

Sadock BJ and Sadock VA. *Kaplan & Sadock's Synopsis of Psychiatry: Behavioral Sciences/Clinical Psychiatry*, 10th edn. Lippincott Williams & Wilkins, 2007, p. 151.

56. E. An immigrant child often tends to conform to the norms of the peer group in his/her host country. Acculturation is the process of behavioural and attitudinal changes as a result of exposure to the practices of a different dominant group, usually seen in people who have immigrated. Children of immigrants born in the host country may achieve a high level of acculturation. The level of acculturation may differ in children born in the host country and those born elsewhere but later migrated to a host country. The degree and nature of the acculturation process is affected by age at immigration, number of years in the host country, language proficiency, and participation in the host culture's social activities, which is likely to be higher in school children, who are in constant contact with their peers, compared to adults.

Martin A and Volkmar FR, eds. *Lewis's Child and Adolescent Psychiatry: A Comprehensive Textbook*, 4th edn. Lippincott Williams & Wilkins, 2007, p. 58.

57. A. Conformity occurs when people yield to real or imagined social pressure. If one listens to rock music in order to avoid being ridiculed by one's friends and not because of one's passion for the music then this exemplifies conformity. The famous Asch's studies in the 1950s provided most experimental background for studying conformity. Asch found that conformity was dependent on group size and group unanimity. People are more likely to conform when they are in ambiguous situations or when they have reasons to doubt their own judgement. Conformity is different from obedience. Obedience follows orders, comes from an authoritative figure, and the subject who obeys usually has no or reduced responsibility compared to the one who makes active decisions.

Thambirajah MS. *Psychological Basis of Psychiatry*. Elsevier, 2005, pp. 204–206.

58. E. Obedience is a form of compliance that occurs when people follow direct commands, usually from someone in a position of authority. Diffusion of personal responsibility, legitimacy of the authority asking one to obey, strong persuasion techniques employed by the authority, and ingrained habit of obeying our parents and teachers as children influence our decision to obey authorities. Social groups depend on a reasonable amount of obedience to function smoothly. In Stanley Milgram's experiment, the 'learners' were never really shocked. In fact the 'teachers' were the real experimental subjects, who believed that a shock was being administered. The "teachers" were asked to deliver the shock by an authoritative 'experimenter'. Milgram's experiments provided some explanations for certain aspects of human behaviour during atrocities such as the Second World War genocides.

Thambirajah MS. *Psychological Basis of Psychiatry*. Elsevier, 2005, p. 207.

59. A. The minority in a social community may feel marginalized when their rights and needs are ignored. Members of the majority may be persuaded or influenced to change their attitude towards the minority by various means in order to reduce conflict between the minority and the majority. In order to achieve this, the minority should present the required message consistently across all the members and through various time intervals. The minority should appear to be acting on principle and making personal sacrifice to become influential within a social group. Age composition or educational status of the minority does not have much effect on the overall influence posed by the minority in a group.

Thambirajah MS. *Psychological Basis of Psychiatry*. Elsevier, 2005, p. 205.

60. D. Deindividuation is a psychological state in which an individual's identity is lost among a collective mass of people and the markers of one's individual personality are conspicuously absent. Anonymity leads to deindividuation and we tend to lose our inhibitions. Deindividuation prevents people from following the prosocial norms of society because they are unidentifiable and therefore feel less pressurized to follow the societal norms. Generally, deindividuation increases aggression unless a group adheres to prescribed codes of practice.

Gross R. *Psychology: The Science of Mind and Behaviour*, 5th edn. Hodder Arnold, 2005, p. 506.

61. A. According to the social facilitation theory, in the presence of others, a dominant response (i.e. a well-learned task) will improve, while a poorly learned response will worsen. For example a well-trained musician would, according to this theory, perform better in the presence of others, but a beginner will make more mistakes. It also depends on the involvement of the audience in the task and on the expectations of praise or criticism.

Thambirajah MS. *Psychological Basis of Psychiatry*. Elsevier, 2005, p. 204.

62. B. The Stages of Change Model by Prochaska and DiClemente are stages that a person goes through when involved in a behavioural change. This may include a change in substance misuse behaviour, starting daily exercise, going on a diet or changing a health-related behaviour, for example attempting to obtain a cervical smear. The first stage is precontemplation stage, where the person is not thinking of any imminent change and is happy the way things are. The second stage is contemplation where he is considering a change in the near future. Preparation is when he gets ready or prepares to make the change. Action phase is where he implements the change and in maintenance phase he decides to continue the change in behaviour and attempts to prevent relapse.

Thambirajah MS. *Psychological Basis of Psychiatry*. Elsevier, 2005, pp. 125–126.

63. B. This observation is otherwise called the bystander apathy or bystander effect. People are less likely to provide help to someone in need if they are in a group rather than when alone. The probability of providing help decreases as the group size increases. One of the main reasons for the bystander effect is diffusion of responsibility, that is a thought that someone else might help. The other influencing factor is the perceived need for help. If it is an emergency situation, we are more likely to intervene and help. Altruism is a different concept and refers to selfless concern about the welfare of others that leads to helping behaviour.

Thambirajah MS. *Psychological Basis of Psychiatry*. Elsevier, 2005, pp. 211–212.

64. C. The reciprocity norm is the situation where you help those who help you. This is a powerful social phenomenon utilized by pharmaceutical representatives. Social responsibility is the situation where you help those in need. Social exchange theory is a theory of interpersonal relationships. It regards relationships in terms similar to trading interactions. According to this theory, a relationship continues as long as both partners feel that the benefits of remaining in the relationship outweigh the costs of the same relationship. According to equity theory, a relationship is successful as long as both partners perceive that the individual outcomes from the relationship are proportional to their individual inputs.

Gross R. *Psychology: The Science of Mind and Behaviour*, 5th edn. Hodder Arnold, 2005, p. 391.
Schetky DH. Conflicts of interest between physicians and the pharmaceutical industry and special interest groups. *Child and Adolescent Psychiatric Clinics of North America* 2008; **17**: 113–125.

65. A. This question tests one's knowledge of Erikson's stages of psychosocial development. Erikson's stages were based on the concept of epigenetic principles. Epigenetic principle states that development occurs in sequential, clearly defined stages, and that each stage must be satisfactorily resolved for development to proceed smoothly. If a stage is not resolved satisfactorily, it results in physical, social, emotional, and cognitive maladjustment. In the question, the lady is 73 years old and is most likely to be in the stage of 'Integrity versus despair', where a person has to resolve the crisis between integrity (feeling at peace with oneself and the world, with no regrets or recriminations) and despair (feeling that life was full of wasted opportunities, regrets, wishing to be able to turn back the clock and have a second chance).

Sadock BJ and Sadock VA. *Kaplan & Sadock's Synopsis of Psychiatry: Behavioral Sciences/Clinical Psychiatry*, 10th edn. Lippincott Williams & Wilkins, 2007, p. 207.

66. D. Short-term memory (referred to by some psychologists as working memory) is a limited capacity store that can maintain unrehearsed information for about 20 to 30 seconds. This duration can be increased by rehearsing. The short-term memory, classically, is also thought to have a capacity of storing seven plus or minus two items. Because of this limited capacity, improving short-term memory storage requires a process called chunking, where identical data are grouped strategically to constitute a single chunk or item. Baddeley proposed an architecture for working memory. According to him, working memory involves three main components: a central executive, two 'slave' systems (the phonological loop and the visuospatial sketch pad), and an episodic buffer. The central executive coordinates the slave systems; the phonological loop contains a phonological store and an articulatory control process and is responsible for inner speech and rehearsing; the visuospatial sketch pad is responsible for setting up and manipulating mental images; the episodic buffer integrates and manipulates material in working memory. A sensory memory store holds a large amount of incoming perceptual information for a very short time, usually a fraction of a second before it can be processed. This store for visual items is called iconic memory and for auditory information is called echoic memory. Sensory memories have a lot of content and are of very brief duration.

Gross R. *Psychology: The Science of Mind and Behaviour*, 5th edn. Hodder Arnold, 2005, pp. 283, 293.

67. A. Procedural memory is a type of memory wherein the knowledge of how to do things (procedures or skills, e.g. swim, ride a bike, typing, etc.) is stored. It may not be conscious. It is not easily communicable and practical demonstration is required. Declarative memory is something we are consciously aware of when we acquire it and we are able to communicate it to another person using language. Episodic memory is a declarative memory for events which can be recalled, for example remembering what one did last summer. It is defined by a specific time scale. Semantic memory is abstract knowledge retained irrespective of how or when it was acquired, for example 'oceans are large bodies of water'. There is no time element attached to semantic memory.

Gross R. *Psychology: The Science of Mind and Behaviour*, 5th edn. Hodder Arnold, 2005, p. 292; Fig. 17.7.

68. A. The serial position effect occurs when people show better recall for items at the beginning and the end of a list compared to those at the middle. This effect includes two components – the primacy effect, which occurs when items near the beginning of the list are recalled better than other items, and the recency effect, which occurs when items at the end are recalled better than other items.

Thambirajah MS. *Psychological Basis of Psychiatry*. Elsevier, 2005, p. 160.

69. D. The stages of a normal male sexual response are desire, excitement, orgasm, and resolution. This is called the DEOR cycle. Traditionally it has also been described as the EPOR cycle, that is excitement, plateau, orgasm, and resolution. Sexual dysfunction can occur due to problems in any of the stages. Depression can lead to a loss of desire. Problems in the excitement phase can lead to erectile dysfunction; problems in the third stage can lead to premature ejaculation.

Sadock BJ and Sadock VA. *Kaplan & Sadock's Synopsis of Psychiatry: Behavioral Sciences/Clinical Psychiatry*, 10th edn. Lippincott Williams & Wilkins, 2007, p. 682.

70. A. According to Maslow, human needs are arranged in a hierarchy. People must satisfy their basic needs before they can satisfy higher needs. Individuals usually progress upwards when their basic needs are relatively satisfied, but may regress back to lower levels. This is especially evident at times of huge natural disasters such as Tsunami or hurricanes. In order of needs, Maslow considered

1. Physiological needs (food, water etc)
2. Safety needs (shelter)
3. Belongingness and love needs
4. Esteem needs
5. Cognitive needs
6. Aesthetic needs
7. Need for self actualization

The latter is the individual's need to fulfill his/her maximum potential. Other therapies as mentioned in the question are pointless when disaster strikes, unless food and shelter needs are met at least partially.

Thambirajah MS. *Psychological Basis of Psychiatry*. Elsevier, 2005, p. 124; see Fig. 5.3

chapter

5

PSYCHOPHARMACOLOGY

QUESTIONS

1. **Aripiprazole is**

   A. A partial agonist at the dopamine receptor
   B. A full agonist at the dopamine receptor
   C. A dopamine receptor antagonist
   D. An inverse agonist
   E. A reuptake inhibitor at the dopamine receptor

2. **Lofexidine is an**

   A. Alpha 2 autoreceptor agonist
   B. Alpha 1 postsynaptic agonist
   C. Alpha 2 autoreceptor antagonist
   D. Alpha 2 heteroceptor agonist
   E. Noradrenaline reuptake inhibitor

3. **Which of the following is NOT a reuptake inhibitor?**

   A. Cocaine
   B. Sertraline
   C. Clomipramine
   D. Bupropion
   E. Buspirone

4. **Which of the following combinations is NOT paired correctly?**

   A. Alprazolam: benzodiazepines
   B. Zopiclone: hypnotics
   C. Haloperidol: butyrophenones
   D. Phenytoin: anticonvulsant
   E. Acamprosate: opiates

5. **Paralytic ileus is most likely to be associated with which one of the following antipsychotics?**

   A. Olanzapine
   B. Haloperidol
   C. Clozapine
   D. Amisulpride
   E. Thioridazine

6. **Which route is most liable for first-pass metabolism?**

    A. Sublingual
    B. Intramuscular
    C. Subcutaneous
    D. Oral
    E. Inhalational

7. **Which of the following statements regarding treatment adherence is FALSE?**

    A. Non-adherence occurs in up to 10% of people with schizophrenia.
    B. Non-adherence increases relapse rate in schizophrenia.
    C. Non-adherence is associated with poor insight.
    D. Adherence is affected by the route of administration.
    E. Adverse effect is a major factor contributing to non-adherence.

8. **If a young male is administered 400 mg of lithium once daily, the average time taken for lithium to reach a steady state in plasma is**

    A. 1 day
    B. 2 days
    C. 10 days
    D. 4 days
    E. 8 days

9. **A 45-year-old man with schizoaffective disorder is on lithium, sertraline, lorazepam, and olanzapine. He develops low sodium levels and complains of extreme lethargy. The most likely offending agent is**

    A. Sertraline
    B. Lithium
    C. Olanzapine
    D. Benzodiazepines
    E. None of the above

10. **Which of the following predisposes to a nocebo effect?**

    A. The expectation of adverse effects at the start of a treatment
    B. Aversive conditioning
    C. Premorbid neuroticism
    D. Coexistent emotional disturbances
    E. All of the above

11. **Flumazenil can reverse the effects of an overdose of which of the following drugs?**

    A. Opioids
    B. Ecstasy (MDMA)
    C. Nitrazepam
    D. Valproate
    E. Clozapine

12. **Regarding depot preparations, which of the following statements is FALSE?**

    A. Depot medications are useful in cases of non-compliance
    B. They undergo less first-pass metabolism than oral preparations
    C. There is less reversibility of side-effects
    D. Injection site reactions are a side-effect
    E. All antipsychotic depot preparations are oil based

13. **Which one of the following is NOT a CYP3A4 inducer?**

    A. St. John's wort
    B. Rifampicin
    C. Barbiturates
    D. Carbamazepine
    E. Fluoxetine

14. **Which of the following statements about first-order kinetics is false?**

    A. A fraction of the drug is eliminated per unit time
    B. Half-life of a drug is directly proportional to the volume of distribution of the drug
    C. Digoxin has a high volume of distribution
    D. Half-life of a drug is directly proportional to the clearance
    E. None of the above

15. **Which of the following is a butyrophenone?**

    A. Risperidone
    B. Quetiapine
    C. Haloperidol
    D. Chlorpromazine
    E. Clozapine

16. **Which of the following medications is NOT associated with zero-order kinetics?**

    A. Phenytoin
    B. Salicylates
    C. Theophylline
    D. Alcohol
    E. Haloperidol

17. **In which of the following situations is a measurement of plasma concentration of a drug the least valuable?**

    A. The drug has a wide therapeutic index
    B. The drug has a therapeutic window
    C. Unexplained toxicity at therapeutic dose
    D. Failure to respond to treatment
    E. Suspected interaction with a co-administered drug

18. **The most probable diagnosis in a clozapine-treated patient who has persistent tachycardia, fatigue, fever, and eosinophilia is:**

   A. Pulmonary embolism
   B. Paralytic ileus
   C. Agranulocytosis
   D. Myocarditis
   E. Atypical NMS

19. **Which of the following patients is at a higher risk of developing lithium-induced hypothyroidism?**

   A. 21-year-old man with bipolar disorder
   B. 33-year-old man with schizoaffective disorder
   C. 45-year-old woman with depression
   D. 14-year-old boy with learning difficulties and aggression
   E. All of the above are at same risk levels

20. **Which one of the following regarding mirtazapine is true? It is**

   A. A central alpha 2 autoreceptor antagonist
   B. A serotonin noradrenalin reuptake inhibitor
   C. A selective serotonin reuptake inhibitor
   D. A tricyclic antidepressant
   E. A dopamine noradrenaline reuptake inhibitor

21. **Which one of the following regarding buspirone is true? It is:**

   A. A tricyclic antidepressant
   B. A selective serotonin reuptake inhibitor
   C. A dopamine antagonist
   D. A partial 5HT agonist
   E. A partial adrenaline agonist

22. **Which of the following drugs stabilizes dopamine release through its action on dopamine receptors?**

   A. Aripiprazole
   B. Quetiapine
   C. Haloperidol
   D. Olanzapine
   E. Chlorpromazine

23. **Which one of the following is NOT a cholinesterase inhibitor?**

   A. Rivastigmine
   B. Donepezil
   C. Gallantamine
   D. Organophosphates
   E. Memantine

24. **Which of the following drugs is NOT metabolized by CYP3A4?**

    A. Clozapine
    B. Quetiapine
    C. Ziprasidone
    D. Sertindole
    E. Risperidone

25. **Select one side-effect of antipsychotics that appears earlier than the others when initiating treatment:**

    A. Tardive dyskinesia
    B. Akathisia
    C. Parkinsonism
    D. Hypothyroidism
    E. Weight gain

26. **Which of the following antidementia drugs is/are prescribed for administration once daily?**

    A. Rivastigmine only
    B. Donepezil only
    C. Gallantamine only
    D. Both rivastigmine and donepezil
    E. Both gallantamine and rivastigmine

27. **The effect of paroxetine on sleep is mainly due to its action on**

    A. $5HT_{1A}$
    B. $5HT_{2A}$
    C. $5HT_3$
    D. Histamine receptors
    E. Cholinergic receptors

28. **Which one of the following is NOT an idiosyncratic reaction?**

    A. Neuroleptic malignant syndrome with antipsychotics
    B. Parkinsonism with antipsychotics
    C. Hepatotoxicity with valproate
    D. Stevens Johnson syndrome with carbamazepine
    E. Rash with lamotrigine

29. **Which of the following is a dose-dependent side-effect?**

    A. Hepatotoxicity due to naltrexone
    B. Agranulocytosis with clozapine
    C. NMS with antipsychotics
    D. Pancreatitis with valproate
    E. Toxic epidermic necrolysis with lamotrigine

30. **Which one of the following affects blood levels of lithium?**
    A. NSAIDS
    B. ACE inhibitors
    C. Thiazide diuretics
    D. Dehydration
    E. All of the above

31. **Which of the following statements is true about plasma levels of clozapine?**
    A. Plasma level monitoring is recommended once weekly for the first 6 months
    B. Plasma levels increase when a smoker stops smoking
    C. In schizophrenia, the recommended plasma level is 150 µg/l
    D. Plasma level is decreased by fluoxetine
    E. None of the above

32. **A 'therapeutic window' is well established in which one of the following?**
    A. Imipramine
    B. Lofepramine
    C. Nortriptyline
    D. Sertraline
    E. Citalopram

33. **A 30-year-old man is started on amitriptyline. He develops dry mouth, constipation, and blurred vision. Action on which of the following receptors could explain the side-effects described?**
    A. Dopamine
    B. Histamine
    C. Muscarinic
    D. Norepinephrine
    E. Serotonin

34. **Which of the following is an example of a pharmacodynamic drug interaction?**
    A. Antacids reduce absorption of chlorpromazine
    B. Valproate displaces warfarin from albumin
    C. Carbamazapine induces the metabolic enzymes
    D. Serotonin syndrome when SSRIs and TCAs are combined
    E. Lithium elimination is decreased by thiazides

35. **Considering psychopharmacology in perinatal psychiatry, which one of the following is true?**
    A. Absolute risk of Ebstein's anomaly in patients treated with lithium is 0.05 to 0.1%
    B. Low-potency, typical antipsychotics are preferred to high-potency drugs
    C. Tricyclic antidepressants should be avoided in pregnancy
    D. SSRIs do not cause neonatal withdrawal syndromes
    E. Animal studies have found no effect of psychotropic medication on brain development and behaviour of the fetus

36. **Which one of the following is NOT a factor affecting the pharmacokinetics of drugs in elderly people?**

   A. Fall in gastric pH
   B. Decreased hepatic blood flow
   C. Reduced glomerular filtration rate
   D. Increased proportion of body fat
   E. Decreased serum albumin

37. **ECT is the first-line treatment for which one of the following?**

   A. Life-threatening depression with refusal of fluid or food
   B. All cases of catatonia
   C. Treatment-resistant schizophrenia
   D. Psychotic depression
   E. Depression with psychomotor retardation

38. **ECT has been found to be useful in which of the following conditions?**

   A. Uncontrolled status epilepticus
   B. On–off phenomena in Parkinson's disease
   C. Neuroleptic malignant syndrome
   D. Hypopituitarism
   E. All of the above

39. **Which of the following is an absolute contraindication for ECT?**

   A. Pregnancy
   B. Intracranial mass
   C. Presence of a metal skull plate
   D. Presence of implanted pacemaker
   E. None of the above

40. **Which of the following statements regarding memory problems associated with ECT is true?**

   A. Amnesia is dependent on the dose of electricity.
   B. Amnesia is not related to electrode placement.
   C. Amnesia for personal events is more common than that for public events.
   D. ECT is commonly followed by persistent anterograde amnesia.
   E. None of the above.

41. **The most common cause for mortality in ECT is**

   A. Fracture of the dorsal vertebrae
   B. Cardiac arrhythmia
   C. Status epilepticus
   D. Herniation of the brain
   E. Electrical burns caused due to poor contact of electrodes

42. **When comparing unilateral and bilateral ECT which of the following is true?**
    A. Memory deficits are less common with bilateral than unilateral ECT
    B. Unilateral ECT is most effective at 2.5 times the seizure threshold
    C. Unilateral ECT is more effective compared to bilateral
    D. Bilateral ECT acts faster than unilateral ECT
    E. Unilateral ECT has better synergistic properties with antidepressants

43. **Which of the following has the shortest plasma half-life?**
    A. Zolpidem
    B. Zaleplon
    C. Zopiclone
    D. Temazepam
    E. Clomethiazole

44. **An elderly gentleman recently started on a hypnotic complains of sneezing and conjunctival irritation. He was most probably started on which of the following drugs?**
    A. Temazepam
    B. Melatonin
    C. Zopiclone
    D. Clomethiazole
    E. Zaleplon

45. **Which of the following is the most potent depot antipsychotic in terms of mg per mg?**
    A. Risperidone long acting
    B. Haloperidol decanoate
    C. Fluphenazine decanoate
    D. Flupentixol decanoate
    E. Pipotiazine palmitate

46. **Which of the following antipsychotics is a drug of choice for a patient with hepatic impairment?**
    A. Risperidone
    B. Amisulpride
    C. Olanzapine
    D. Quetiapine
    E. Aripiprazole

47. **Which of the following antipsychotics has the LEAST effect on weight gain?**
    A. Aripiprazole
    B. Olanzapine
    C. Quetiapine
    D. Risperidone
    E. Clozapine

48. **Which of the following is a dibenzothiazepine in its chemical structure?**
    A. Risperidone
    B. Clozapine
    C. Olanzapine
    D. Quetiapine
    E. Amisulpride

49. **Which of the following is true about tardive dyskinesia?**
    A. Develops in up to 50% of patients treated with schizophrenia
    B. Risk factor include being a young male with a history of mood disorder
    C. TD is said to be due to the down regulation of dopamine receptors
    D. Stopping the antipsychotics worsens TD temporarily
    E. Anticholinergics such as procyclidine are the treatment of choice

50. **Which of the following drugs has the greatest effect on QTc interval?**
    A. Quetiapine
    B. Thioridazine
    C. Olanzapine
    D. Aripiprazole
    E. Risperidone

51. **Which of the following is potentially antagonistic at dopamine receptors?**
    A. Imipramine
    B. Clomipramine
    C. Amoxapine
    D. Amitriptyline
    E. Nortriptyline

52. **Which of the following tricyclic antidepressants is the preferred drug compared to the others listed when prescribed to a patient with cardiovascular illness?**
    A. Imipramine
    B. Clomipramine
    C. Lofepramine
    D. Amitriptyline
    E. Nortriptyline

53. **Which of the following is more common with SSRIs compared to TCAs?**
    A. Switch to mania
    B. Seizures
    C. Parkinsonian side-effects
    D. Cardiac side-effects
    E. None of the above

54. **Serotonin syndrome is possible when SSRIs are combined with which of the following?**

    A. Lithium
    B. MAOIs
    C. Sumatriptan
    D. Tryptophan
    E. All of the above

55. **In a patient with depression, an SSRI would be the drug of choice, EXCEPT when**

    A. The patient has concomitant cardiac disease
    B. Sedation is desired
    C. There is a risk of overdose
    D. History of intolerance to anticholinergic side-effects
    E. Depression is associated with obsessive compulsive symptoms

56. **Which of the following statements regarding drug interactions is true?**

    A. Salbutamol inhalers are safe in patients taking MAOIs.
    B. Combining MAOIs and tricyclics could lead to severe postural hypotension.
    C. MAOIs are sedating at therapeutic doses.
    D. Moclobemide is not associated with tyramine reaction.
    E. Incidence of hypertensive reaction in patients on MAOIs is less than 1%.

57. **Which of the following is associated with leucocytosis?**

    A. Clozapine
    B. Mianserin
    C. Mirtazapine
    D. Lithium
    E. Carbamazepine

58. **Which of the following is true with regard to lamotrigine?**

    A. Valproate decreases levels of lamotrigine
    B. Carbamazepine increases the level of lamotrigine
    C. Lamotrigine monotherapy has been found to be effective in bipolar mania
    D. Lamotrigine induces cytochrome enzymes
    E. Lamotrigine blocks voltage-dependent sodium channels

59. **Which of the following is associated with inappropriate secretion of antidiuretic hormone (SIADH)?**

    A. Fluoxetine
    B. Venlafaxine
    C. Haloperidol
    D. Amitriptyline
    E. All of the above

60. **Which of the following is LESS likely to cause a discontinuation reaction than others in the list?**

A. Venlafaxine
B. Fluoxetine
C. Paroxetine
D. Citalopram
E. Amitriptyline

1. A. When a neurotransmitter has a stimulating effect on receptors, this leads to agonistic actions. Drugs which stimulate receptors similar to these neurotransmitters are therefore called agonists. Drugs which block the action of the neurotransmitter on the receptors are antagonists. They act only in the presence of the neurotransmitter and do not have any intrinsic activity on their own. Inverse agonists have the opposite action of an agonist. For example, instead of opening an agonist operated channel, they close the channel after binding to the receptor. Inverse agonists thus have intrinsic activity (can act even in the absence of neurotransmitter molecules in the vicinity) and so can also be blocked by the antagonist. Partial agonists act as net agonists in the absence of the neurotransmitter, but act as a net antagonist in the presence of the neurotransmitter. Aripiprazole is a partial agonist at the dopamine (D_2) receptor.

Gelder MG *et al.*, eds. *Shorter Oxford Textbook of Psychiatry*, 5th edn. Oxford University Press, 2006, p. 532.

2. A. Lofexidine is an alpha 2 agonist which acts at the autoreceptor. When the presynaptic autoreceptors are stimulated, they generally stop the release of the particular neurotransmitter. Thus they act as a brake. Lofexidine stimulates the alpha 2 autoreceptors, thus stopping the release of noradrenaline into the synapse. The antagonists of autoreceptors increase the release of the neurotransmitter. In the case of serotonin, $5HT_{1B}$ are autoreceptors. Some alpha 2 receptors are found on serotonergic neurones and control the release of 5HT; these alpha 2 receptors are called heteroreceptors.

Gelder MG *et al.*, eds. *Shorter Oxford Textbook of Psychiatry*, 5th edn. Oxford University Press, 2006, p. 459.

3. E. Buspirone is a partial agonist at $5\text{-}HT_{1A}$ autoreceptors and can influence the firing of serotonergic (5-HT) neurones. Neurotransmitters in the synaptic cleft are actively transported back into the presynaptic neurone by a reuptake pump. Most antidepressants block this pump, thus increasing the availability of the monoamine neurotransmitters. Cocaine is a dopamine reuptake inhibitor. Bupropion inhibits reuptake of both dopamine and noradrenaline.

Gelder MG *et al.*, eds. *New Oxford Textbook of Psychiatry*. Oxford University Press, 2000, pp. 1279–1281.

4. E. Phenytoin is an anticonvulsant. Alprazolam is a benzodiazepine and it is not used as a mood stabilizer; valproate, lithium, lamotrigine, and carbamazepine can be considered as mood stabilizers. Haloperidol is a butyrophenone and not a phenothiazine. Acamprosate is used to treat alcohol dependence. It is not an opiate. It has a structure similar to GABA and it is thought to act via glutamate receptor mechanism. Zopiclone is not a benzodiazepine. It is a hypnotic classed with other 'Z drugs'; Z drugs are non-benzodiazepines which act on the GABA complex but at a slightly different site than benzodiazepines.

Sadock BJ and Sadock VA. *Kaplan & Sadock's Synopsis of Psychiatry: Behavioral Sciences/Clinical Psychiatry*, 10th edn. Lippincott Williams & Wilkins, 2007, p. 1018.

5. C.   Clozapine causes anticholinergic effects by blocking muscarinic (M3) receptors. This can cause side-effects such as dry mouth, constipation, loss of accommodation, and urinary retention. Constipation is a side-effect in around 15% of patients taking clozapine, and, in most, simple advice about diet and fluid intake is sufficient. More significant ileus is an uncommon but potentially more serious side-effect. It may particularly be associated with bowel surgery. It could potentially be fatal. Though isolated reports of similar problems with olanzapine and risperidone have been recorded, these are not well-established associations.

Taylor D et al., eds. The Maudsley Prescribing Guidelines, 8th edn. Taylor and Francis, 2005, p. 54.

6. D.   Orally administered drugs reach the liver via the portal circulation. If hepatic metabolism is extensive, a large amount of drug will be removed during this first passage through the liver. Thus, even if a drug is extensively absorbed, first-pass removal will reduce its systemic availability. So, drugs administered parenterally may need lower dosage compared to the same compound taken orally. Apart from the liver, first pass metabolism also takes place in gut mucosa, muscle tissue, and lung parenchyma, albeit to a smaller extent.

Gelder MG et al., eds. New Oxford Textbook of Psychiatry. Oxford University Press, 2000, p. 1278.

7. A.   Non-adherence occurs in up to 40–60% of patients with schizophrenia at any time. Adherence is a multidimensional and dynamic concept and it is not useful to consider adherence vs non-adherence as the only categories in the spectrum. Non-adherence is not exclusive to psychosis; it has also been recorded in other psychiatric disorders including depression. In fact, adherence is a problem even in non-psychiatric but long-term illnesses such as diabetes and hypertension. Side-effects are major factors in causing non-adherence. Depot preparations have better adherence rates, largely due to direct supervision and non-reversibility.

Lacro JP, et al. Prevalence of and risk factors for medication non adherence in patients with schizophrenia: a comprehensive review of recent literature. Journal of Clinical Psychiatry 2002; **63**: 892–909.

8. D.   The time taken for a drug to reach the steady state is the function of its half-life. If the drug is given regularly within its half-life, it will reach a steady state in the plasma in about four to five half-lives. In this case, Lithium has a half-life of nearly 24 hours. So if we give lithium once daily for 4 days, it would have reached a steady state, and a blood taken on the 4th or 5th morning 12 hours after the last dose will give the trough lithium level, which will be an estimate of the plasma level of lithium.

Gelder MG et al., eds. New Oxford Textbook of Psychiatry. Oxford University Press, 2000, p. 1279.

9. A.   Hyponatraemia has a well-known association with the use of antidepressants, especially SSRIs. Elderly people and those medically frail are worst affected. Hyponatraemia can also confuse the picture of depression by inducing lethargy and fatigue. The propensity to cause hyponatraemia seems to be a class effect of antidepressants – so replacing an SSRI with another SSRI will not eliminate the risk completely. Carbamazepine is also associated with SIADH and hyponatraemia. Lithium causes nephrogenic diabetes insipidus and sodium levels are either normal or marginally high as a result. Antipsychotics are also reported to be associated with hyponatraemia, although SSRIs are more likely to be associated with this phenomenon.

Taylor et al., eds. The Maudsley Prescribing Guidelines, 8th edn. Taylor and Francis, 2005, p. 159.

10. E. Placebos can also have adverse effects. Some patients will not tolerate placebos despite the fact that they are inert, and suffer from adverse effects (called the nocebo phenomenon). Nocebo effects with medication include all complaints mistakenly attributed to the medication, such as symptoms of the illness itself, symptoms of stress and the emotional response thereto, symptoms that reflect the patient's normal physiology, and symptoms that reflect normal variations in health. Predisposing factors for a nocebo response include expectations of adverse effects at the onset of treatment, conditioning, wherein the patient learns from prior experiences to associate medication taking with certain somatic symptoms, predisposition due to gender (women complain more), neuroticism, hypochondriasis, a tendency to somatize, coexistent emotional disturbances, and situational and contextual factors that alter expectations or result in aversive conditioning.

Barsky AJ, Saintfort R, Rogers MP, and Borus JF. Nonspecific medication side effects and the nocebo phenomenon. *Journal of the American Medical Association* 2002; **287**: 622–627.

11. C. Flumazenil is an antagonist of benzodiazepine receptors at the GABA$_A$ complex. It is used to reverse sedative effects of benzodiazepines used in anaesthesia and in management of benzodiazepine overdose. As a result of this effect, it can precipitate benzodiazepine withdrawal seizures and can also precipitate anxiety in patients with anxiety/ panic disorder. It is not used to treat benzodiazepine withdrawal symptoms. It is not useful for any other drug toxicity or abuse as mentioned in the question. Naloxone is used in opioid overdose.

Taylor *et al.*, eds. *The Maudsley Prescribing Guidelines*, 8th edn. Taylor and Francis, 2005, p. 317

12. E. Depot antipsychotic drugs have the following advantages: they decrease the risk of problems associated with medication non-compliance and undergo significantly less first-pass metabolism. The disadvantages include the fact that, once injected, the drug cannot be removed and hence adverse effects or adverse drug interactions are less reversible. An associated complication is injection site reaction. Depot risperidone is an aqueous suspension of risperidone in a glycolic acid–lactate copolymer matrix. The copolymer is slowly hydrolysed, resulting in the gradual release of risperidone. As depot risperidone is water based, it causes fewer reactions than the other oil-based preparations.

Grant S and Fitton A. Risperidone: a review of its pharmacology and therapeutic potential in the treatment of schizophrenia. *Drugs* 1994; **48**: 253–273.

13. E. Fluoxetine is an inhibitor of CYP450 enzymes. CYP1A2 is inhibited by fluvoxamine and duloxetine, and induced by phenytoin. CYP2D6 is inhibited by fluoxetine, paroxetine, sertraline, and duloxetine. CYP3A4 is inhibited by fluoxetine, nefazodone, and sertraline and is induced by carbamazepine, phenobarbital, and phenytoin. CYP2C9/10/19 is inhibited by fluvoxamine, fluoxetine, moclobemide, sertraline, and minimally by venlafaxine. St John's wort induces CYP3A4. CYP3A4 metabolizes carbamazepine, oral contraceptives, atypical antipsychotics, Z hypnotics, benzodiazepines, and calcium channel blockers.

Taylor *et al.*, eds. *The Maudsley Prescribing Guidelines*, 8th edn. Taylor and Francis, 2005, p. 180

14. D. In first order kinetics, a constant fraction of the drug in the body is eliminated per unit time. The rate of elimination is proportional to the amount of drug in the body. The majority of psychiatric drugs are eliminated in this way. Volume of distribution is the amount of drug in the body divided by the concentration in the blood. So a drug that is highly lipid soluble and redistributes into fat has a high volume of distribution (Vd). These drugs stay out of the blood most of the time and, as a result, will have a long half-life. The lesser the clearance of the drug, the longer the half-life; so half-life is inversely proportional to the clearance. Digoxin is highly lipid soluble and has a long half-life.

Gelder MG *et al.*, eds. *New Oxford Textbook of Psychiatry*. Oxford University Press, 2000, p. 1287.

15. C. Risperidone is a benzisoxazole; quetiapine is a dibenzothiazepine; clozapine and is a dibenzodiazepines; olanzapine is a thienobenzodiazepine; sulpiride and amisulpiride are substituted benzamides; chlorpromazine is a phenothazine; and haloperidol is a butyrophenone.

Johnstone EC et al., eds. *Companion to Psychiatric Studies*, 7th edn. Churchill Livingstone, 2004, p. 259.

16. E. Zero-order kinetics occurs when the body metabolizes a constant amount of the drug. The metabolic pathway is rapidly saturated, leading to a limit being set for drug elimination. So only a constant amount of drug is eliminated irrespective of plasma levels, for example our body can metabolize around 1 unit of alcohol per hour; if you have taken 4 units, it will take 4 hours for the alcohol to get out of your system. So the time taken is directly proportional to the amount consumed, unlike in first-order kinetics where it takes four to five half-lives for the drug to get out of the system, irrespective of the dose consumed. The most important difference to remember is that a constant fraction (percentage) is eliminated in first-order kinetics while a constant amount is eliminated in zero-order kinetics.

Gelder MG et al., eds. *New Oxford Textbook of Psychiatry*. Oxford University Press, 2000, p. 1287.

17. A. Measurement of plasma level is not routinely done for most of the available psychotropic medications. But it is useful, and often indicated, when there is a therapeutic window, suspected drug interactions, unusual toxic reaction at therapeutic doses, and non-response to treatment in spite of administering adequate dose. Therapeutic window is a range of plasma concentration within which a drug produces the therapeutic response. If the level of drug is outside the defined 'window', the therapeutic response is inadequate. Therapeutic index is a ratio of median toxic dose to median effective dose of a drug. Failure to respond to treatment may be due to non-compliance, which can be detected in some cases by measuring the plasma levels.

Sadock BJ and Sadock VA. *Kaplan & Sadock's Synopsis of Psychiatry: Behavioral Sciences/Clinical Psychiatry*, 10th edn. Lippincott Williams & Wilkins, 2007, p. 986.

18. D. Myocarditis is a fatal complication of clozapine use. It can occur very subtly with observable signs developing well after cardiac failure sets in. This is an idiosyncratic, eosinophilic inflammation of the myocardium. Persistent tachycardia, fever (flu like), chest pain, palpitations, dependent oedema, and signs of heart failure must prompt a detailed investigation, including cardiac enzymes (elevated), ECG (ST elevation), ESR (elevated), WBC (eosinophilia), and echocardiogram. With a good monitoring system in place for agranulocytosis, myocarditis is becoming a leading cause of clozapine-related fatalities.

Taylor et al., eds. *The Maudsley Prescribing Guidelines*, 8th edn. Taylor and Francis, 2005, p. 58.

19. C. It is well established that the risk of hypothyroidism related to lithium use varies widely across the population. Middle-aged women, who probably have a higher risk of having asymptomatic antithyroid antibodies before initiation of lithium, are at the maximum risk of clinical hypothyroidism (up to 20% prevalence). Importantly, this hypothyroidism does not correlate with the dose of lithium prescribed.

Taylor et al., eds. *The Maudsley Prescribing Guidelines*, 8th edn. Taylor and Francis, 2005, p. 113.

20. A. Mirtazapine is called a noradrenergic and specific serotonergic antidepressant (NaSSA). The therapeutic action of mirtazapine is due to central alpha 2 antagonist action, thus cutting the brakes for the release of norepinephrine (alpha 2 inhibitory autoreceptors) and serotonin (alpha 2 heteroreceptors constantly inhibit serotonin release too). Mirtazapine also acts as an antagonist at $5HT_{2A}$, $5HT_{2C}$, and $5HT_3$ receptors, which may contribute to the favourable side-effect profile compared to SSRIs. Mianserin acts in a similar way. Mirtazapine does not block the reuptake pump.

Stahl SM. *Essential Psychopharmacology: Neuroscientific Basis and Practical Application*, 2nd edn. Cambridge University Press, 2000, p. 253.

21. D. Buspirone is a partial agonist at $5HT_{1A}$. It is used in generalized anxiety disorder and as an augmenting agent to treat resistant depression. It does not have an action on the GABA receptors; hence it is free from interaction with alcohol and benzodiazepines. It does not lead to dependence or withdrawal symptoms with long-term use. It has a delayed onset of action similar to antidepressants.

Stahl SM. *Essential Psychopharmacology: Neuroscientific Basis and Practical Application*, 2nd edn. Cambridge University Press, 2000, p. 273.

22. A. Aripiprazole has been dubbed a dopamine system stabilizer due to its partial agonist action. It acts as an agonist where dopamine is depleted and acts as an antagonist where there is an excess of dopamine, making the availability of dopamine 'just right' for normal function.

Stahl SM. Dopamine system stabilizers, aripiprazole, and the next generation of antipsychotics, part 1, 'Goldilocks' actions at dopamine receptors. *Journal of Clinical Psychiatry* 2001; **62**: 841–842.

23. E. Memantine acts by partially blocking NMDA receptors, thereby preventing cell death related to calcium-mediated excitotoxicity. Donepezil is a non-competitive, reversible acetyl cholinesterase inhibitor (AChI). Rivastigmine is a non-competitive inhibitor for both butyryl cholinesterase and acetyl cholinesterase. Gallantamine is a competitive, reversible inhibitor which modulates nicotinic receptors. Tacrine is a non-competitive, non-selective, reversible inhibitor which acts both centrally and peripherally. It is no longer used because of high hepatotoxicity. Organophosphates are often used in pesticides and have acetyl cholinesterase-inhibiting properties.

Sadock BJ and Sadock VA. *Kaplan & Sadock's Synopsis of Psychiatry: Behavioral Sciences/Clinical Psychiatry*, 10th edn. Lippincott Williams & Wilkins, 2007, p. 1033.

24. E. Among the antipsychotics, typical antipsychotics are mostly metabolized through CYP2D6. Risperidone is metabolized by CYP2D6. Clozapine and olanzapine are primarily metabolized through CYP1A2, and to a lesser extent, through the CYP 3A4 enzyme system. Olanzapine is also metabolized through the CYP3A4 enzyme system. The other antipsychotics listed in Question 24 are metabolized through the CYP3A4 system.

Gelder MG *et al.*, eds. *Shorter Oxford Textbook of Psychiatry*, 5th edn. Oxford University Press, 2006, p. 547.

25. B. Akathisia occurs within hours to days after onset of antipsychotic treatment in most vulnerable cases. Prevalence is thought to be around 25%. It has both a subjective component of inner restlessness and an objective motor restlessness, manifested as constant pacing, shuffling, or inability to stand still. A specific rating scale to measure akathisia is the Barnes Akathisia Rating Scale. It is to be distinguished from psychotic agitation as akathisia has been linked to suicide and violence. Akathisia can also be caused by serotonergic antidepressants that stimulate $5HT_2$ receptors. A slow-developing form of akathisia, called tardive akathisia, may be particularly difficult to treat. There is also some evidence to say that persistent akathisia (especially the tardive variant) may predict the development of tardive dyskinesia in the future. Dystonic reactions can occur within minutes of administration of injectable antipsychotics in vulnerable individuals. They are less common with the atypical antipsychotics compared to highly potent, typical antipsychotics (prevalence 10%).

Taylor *et al.*, eds. *The Maudsley Prescribing Guidelines*, 8th edn. Taylor and Francis, 2005, p. 76.

26. B. Donepezil is administered once daily. This is possible because of the extended half-life of donepezil compared to other antidementia drugs. Gallantamine and rivastigmine are administered twice daily. An extended release form of gallantamine is now available and this can be administered once daily.

Sadock BJ and Sadock VA. *Kaplan & Sadock's Synopsis of Psychiatry: Behavioral Sciences/Clinical Psychiatry*, 10th edn. Lippincott Williams & Wilkins, 2007, p. 1035.

27. B. Unlike tricyclic antidepressants, most SSRIs have a disruptive effect on sleep, hence administered in the morning. Stimulation of serotonin $5HT_{2A}$ receptors in the brainstem sleep centres may cause rapid muscle movements called myoclonus during the night; it may also disrupt slow-wave sleep and cause nocturnal awakenings. $5 HT_{2A}$ and $5HT_{2C}$ are also responsible for the panic attacks and anxiety associated with SSRIs. $5HT_3$ receptors are involved in the gastrointestinal side-effects like nausea and vomiting, mediated through their location at the chemoreceptor trigger zone. SSRIs generally have very much less or absent antihistamine or anticholinergic action, except paroxetine which has significant anticholinergic activity. The antidepressant action of SSRIs is thought to be mediated through the down-regulation of $5HT_{1A}$ autoreceptors.

Stahl SM. *Essential Psychopharmacology: Neuroscientific Basis and Practical Application*, 2nd edn. Cambridge University Press, 2000, p. 233

28. B. Side-effects are generally divided into two types. Dose-dependent side-effects can be predicted, for example postural hypotension or parkinsonian side-effects with antipsychotics. Dose-independent side-effects are either idiosyncratic or immune-mediated side-effects that cannot be predicted in a patient beforehand, for example anaphylactic reactions. Lamotrigine-induced rash is dose independent and often occurs during the early phase of treatment. Hepatotoxicity due to valproate and Steven Johnson syndrome related to carbamazepine are potentially life-threatening, idiosyncratic effects.

Gelder MG *et al.*, eds. *New Oxford Textbook of Psychiatry*. Oxford University Press, 2000, p. 1282; Table 3.

29. A. Agranulocytosis can occur at any given dose of clozapine. It is not a dose-dependent effect. The risk of agranulocytosis is higher in the first year of clozapine therapy and gradually reduces over the course of treatment. Similarly, neuroleptic malignant syndrome is an idiosyncratic reaction which cannot be predicted in an individual patient. The most important clinical implication to remember is the fact that if a patient has an idiosyncratic side-effect, then this can reoccur at even small doses if rechallenged. Stopping the drug rather than lowering its dose is the appropriate management strategy in such cases. Naltrexone produces hepatocellular damage in proportion to the dose administered, especially in patients with pre-existing liver damage.

Gelder MG *et al.*, eds. *New Oxford Textbook of Psychiatry*. Oxford University Press, 2000, p. 1282; Table 3.

30. E. The clearance of lithium is delayed by most non-steroidal anti-inflammatory drugs including cyclo-oxygenase 2 (COX-2) inhibitors. Thiazide diuretics increase the plasma concentration of lithium. Other drugs which increase the concentration of lithium include ACE inhibitors. SSRIs increase the risk of serotonin syndrome with lithium, while haloperidol and carbamazepine increase the risk of neurotoxicity without altering plasma levels.

Taylor *et al.*, eds. *The Maudsley Prescribing Guidelines*, 8th edn. Taylor and Francis, 2005, p. 114.

31. B. Clozapine plasma level monitoring is indicated in patients who are not responding to standard doses of clozapine. A plasma level of 350 µg/l is reasonable for most patients. A full blood count is done initially weekly while starting clozapine, in accordance with the clozapine patient monitoring service guidelines. Smoking induces the enzymes that metabolize clozapine. Hence, stopping smoking can increase the levels of clozapine. Fluoxetine is an inhibitor of CYP1A2, which metabolizes clozapine and may increase the levels of clozapine. This may also be therapeutic at times, in patients who do not respond to a maximum dose of clozapine.

Taylor *et al.*, eds. *The Maudsley Prescribing Guidelines*, 8th edn. Taylor and Francis, 2005, p. 47.

32. C. A therapeutic window is a range of concentrations of a drug measured in the blood that are associated with a good therapeutic response. Plasma concentrations outside this range are either too low to ensure a therapeutic response or so high that they induce toxic side-effects. There is no evidence to say that there is an established therapeutic window for neuroleptics. Lithium has a therapeutic window. Nortriptyline is the only medication in the list that appears to have an established therapeutic window, in the range of 50 to 150 ng/ml. This level is usually reached by doses ranging from 50 to 100 mg/day.

Leonard BE. *Fundamentals of Psychopharmacology*, 3rd edn. Wiley, 2003, p. 81.

33. C. The side-effects mentioned in the question are features suggestive of the action of the tricyclic antidepressant on muscarinic cholinergic receptors. This includes dry mouth, urinary retention, blurred vision, and constipation. Dry mouth may lead to caries teeth in the long term. In the case of overdose with TCA, the anticholinergic action can lead to confusion, coma, and death due to respiratory failure. Action on α-adrenoceptors, may result in postural hypotension, causing falls and injuries. Therapeutic action of TCAs is thought to be due to its inhibitor action on serotonin and norepinephrine reuptake pumps. Amoxapine is a tricyclic antidepressant of the dibenzoxazepine class, which has a dopamine receptor blocking effect. Amoxapine may be useful in cases of psychotic depression due to its dopamine blocking properties.

Henry JA. Toxicity of newer versus older antidepressants. *Advances in Psychiatric Treatment* 1997; **3**: 41–45.

34. D. There are two main types of drug interactions, pharmacodynamic and pharmacokinetic. Pharmacodynamic interactions arise when one drug increases or decreases the pharmacological effect of a second drug that is given at the same time, for example the depressant action of alcohol is augmented by benzodiazepines. When one drug alters a pharmacokinetic component of another drug, thus causing a change in the concentration of the other drug, this is called a pharmacokinetic interaction, for example inhibition of CYP450 enzyme, displacement of a drug from protein binding, reduced renal excretion of a drug, etc.

Gelder MG *et al.*, eds. *Shorter Oxford Textbook of Psychiatry*, 5th edn. Oxford University Press, 2006, p. 521.

35. A. Most psychotropic medications are best avoided in the first trimester. Caution should also be exercised at the time of delivery and early neonatal period. Most medications, including lithium, are secreted in breast milk and should be used with caution. TCAs and fluoxetine have the best evidence for safety in pregnancy. Lithium can cause Ebstein's anomaly (cardiac valvular deformity) and floppy baby syndrome in newborns. SSRI withdrawal may be seen in newborns, especially if the mother was on short-acting SSRIs immediately prior to delivery. With respect to antipsychotics, high potency drugs are preferred to low potency ones in pregnancy. Anticonvulsant mood stabilizers have a high risk of neural tube defects. Benzodiazepines have a high risk of cleft lip.

Gelder MG *et al.*, eds. *Shorter Oxford Textbook of Psychiatry*, 5th edn. Oxford University Press, 2006, p. 523.

36. A. Gut motility and acid secretion decrease with age. Elderly people have more fat relative to muscle mass, less water, and less body protein than younger adults. This leads to an increase in volume of distribution and longer half-life of administered drugs; 35% of renal function is lost by 65 years of age. Gastric pH increases (not decreases, as indicated in the question) due to loss of acidity.

Semple DM *et al.*, eds. *Oxford Handbook of Psychiatry*, 1st edn. Oxford University Press, 2005, p. 486.

Taylor *et al.*, eds. *The Maudsley Prescribing Guidelines*, 8th edn. Taylor and Francis, 2005, p. 299.

37. A. All of the given options may are considered as indications for ECT. But according to the Royal College of Psychiatrists and NICE (UK), ECT as a first-line treatment of choice must be restricted to suicidal patients and those whose illness is life threatening due to refusal of food and fluids.

National Institute for Clinical Excellence. *Guidance in the Use of Electroconvulsive Therapy* (Technology Appraisal Guidance 59). London: NICE, 2003.

38. E. ECT has been found to be useful in some physical conditions, including those listed in the question, as well as symptoms associated with tardive dystonia.

Sadock BJ and Sadock VA. *Kaplan & Sadock's Synopsis of Psychiatry: Behavioral Sciences/Clinical Psychiatry*, 10th edn. Lippincott Williams & Wilkins, 2007, p. 1120.

39. E. There are no absolute contraindications for ECT. All the known contraindications are relative. Any medical illness that could compromise the patient's status under general anaesthesia is considered a relative contraindication. ECT has been reported to be safe in people with pacemakers and metal skull plates, though caution is needed. ECT is safe in pregnancy and is a preferred treatment in depressed, pregnant patients with a high risk to self or the baby.

Sadock BJ and Sadock VA. *Kaplan & Sadock's Synopsis of Psychiatry: Behavioral Sciences/Clinical Psychiatry*, 10th edn. Lippincott Williams & Wilkins, 2007, p. 1120.

40. A. Amnesia is dependent on the dose of electricity that exceeds the threshold stimulus needed to elicit a seizure in a given patient. The higher the dose, the greater the memory disturbance. It is also dependent on the electrode placement and more severe with bilateral placement than unilateral. Remote memory loss for impersonal/ public events is more common than amnesia for personal events. ECT is rarely followed by persistent anterograde amnesia.

Gelder MG *et al.*, eds. *Shorter Oxford Textbook of Psychiatry*, 5th edn. Oxford University Press, 2006, p. 568.

41. B. Mortality with ECT is about the same as that with general anaesthesia for any minor surgery. The American Psychiatric Association Task Force on ECT estimated that the ECT-related mortality rate is 1 in 10,000 patients or 1 in 80,000 treatments. ECT is considered a low-risk procedure, even in an elderly cardiac patient who, in the developed world, is fast becoming the modal candidate for ECT. It is noted that ECT is about 10 times safer than childbirth and, each year, approximately six times as many deaths in the USA are caused by lightning than by ECT. In those who die, the commonest cause is a cardiac event, usually an arrhythmia.

Abrams R. The mortality rate with ECT. *Convulsive Therapy* 1997; **13**: 125–127.

42. D. Overall, bilateral ECT has superior efficacy compared to unilateral, although bilateral is associated with more side-effects. Recent studies have shown that high-dose unilateral is better than low-dose bilateral in terms of side-effects and equivalent in terms of efficacy. When choosing right unilateral placement, a higher dose titration is preferred. If there is a need for urgent improvement, bilateral placement is recommended.

Gelder MG *et al.*, eds. *Shorter Oxford Textbook of Psychiatry*, 5th edn. Oxford University Press, 2006, p. 567.

43. B. Z hypnotics are non-benzodiazepines which act at or close to the benzodiazepine receptor site in the GABA$_A$ complex. Its action is reversed by flumazenil. Zaleplon has the shortest half-life (1 hour) among the sedatives listed in the question. Temazepam (5–11 hours) and clomethiazole (4–6 hours) are also used as hypnotics. They are usually prescribed short term for the induction of sleep, usually for not more than 2 weeks.

Gelder MG *et al.*, eds. *Shorter Oxford Textbook of Psychiatry*, 5th edn. Oxford University Press, 2006, p. 529.

44. D. Clomethiazole is a hypnotic with anticonvulsant properties. It causes dependence and respiratory depression with alcohol. It is used in elderly people because of its relatively shorter half-life. Unwanted side-effects include sneezing, conjunctival irritation, and nausea.

Gelder MG *et al.*, eds. *Shorter Oxford Textbook of Psychiatry*, 5th edn. Oxford University Press, 2006, p. 530.

45. E. Pipothiazine is the most potent in terms of dose–response of the depot neuroleptics; 5 mg of pipothiazine is equivalent to: 100 mg of haloperidol, 25 mg of risperidone, 25 mg of fluphenazine, 40 mg of flupentixol, and 200 mg of zuclopenthixol.

Gelder MG *et al.*, eds. *Shorter Oxford Textbook of Psychiatry*, 5th edn. Oxford University Press, 2006, p. 533.

46. B. Most antipsychotics, with the notable exception of amisulpiride, are highly lipid soluble and extensively metabolized by the liver. Amisulpiride is excreted unchanged by the kidney. Amisulpride is also considered unique in that it is a highly selective dopamine D2/D3 receptor antagonist that binds preferentially to receptors in the mesolimbic system. It is also an 'atypical' antipsychotic despite, having a different receptor-affinity profile compared to the other atypical antipsychotics (i.e. absence of serotonin antagonism). At low doses (50 mg), amisulpride preferentially blocks presynaptic autoreceptors, producing an increase in dopamine release, leading to some amelioration of the dopaminergic hypoactivity seen in negative symptoms of schizophrenia and depression. At higher doses (400–1200 mg), the drug exerts its activity on postsynaptic D_3/D_2 receptors located in the limbic region and prefrontal areas, producing selective dopaminergic inhibition.

Gelder MG *et al.*, eds. *Shorter Oxford Textbook of Psychiatry*, 5th edn. Oxford University Press, 2006, p. 533.

47. A. Clozapine and olanzapine produce the maximum weight gain among antipsychotics. Aripiprazole is considered to be weight neutral, according to the currently available data. Ziprasidone, which is not marketed in the UK, is said to be associated with some weight loss. Average increases reported during the first year are 5.3 to 6.3 kg for clozapine and 6.8 to 11.8 kg for olanzapine, with some subgroups gaining more than 20% of their initial body weight. Moreover, Leiberman *et al.*, found that weight gain appears to be a continuous process where no relationship exists between the dose of antipsychotics prescribed and degree of weight gain.

Gelder MG *et al.*, eds. *Shorter Oxford Textbook of Psychiatry*, 5th edn. Oxford University Press, 2006, p. 532.

Lieberman JA, Stroup TS, McEvoy JP, *et al.* Effectiveness of antipsychotic drugs in patients with chronic schizophrenia. *New England Journal of Medicine* 2005; **353**: 1209–1223.

48. D. Quetiapine is a dibenzothiazepine. It acts similar to clozapine; both drugs having a 'hit-and-run' profile on D_2 receptors. Quetiapine does not stay at the receptor site for a long time to produce extrapyramidal effects but instead it produces a transient blockade. This has been demonstrated using 11C Raclopride PET studies.

Gelder MG *et al.*, eds. *Shorter Oxford Textbook of Psychiatry*, 5th edn. Oxford University Press, 2006, p. 531.

Kapur S, Zipursky RB *et al.* A positron emission tomography study of quetiapine in schizophrenia: a preliminary finding of an antipsychotic effect with only transiently high dopamine D2 receptor occupancy. *Archives of General Psychiatry* 2000; **57**: 553–559.

49. D. In tardive dyskinesia (TD) the movements can be choreiform, athetoid, dystonic, stereotypic, or a combination of these. They most commonly involve the orobuccal, lingual, and facial muscles. High risk groups includes women, elderly, patients with underlying brain damage, those with mood disorder or schizoaffective illness, learning disability, and, curiously, patients with diabetes. It is seen in up to 20% of people on long-term antipsychotic medications. The pathophysiology behind TD is considered to be receptor up-regulation (increase in postsynaptic receptor numbers due to chronic pharmacological antagonism). So, increasing the dose of the offending drugs may suppress the dyskinetic movements for a short while. Anticholinergic drugs, on the other hand, may aggravate TD. Strategies for the management of tardive dyskinesia include gradual withdrawal of antipsychotic medication, a switch to clozapine, and discontinuation of the anticholinergic medication. Tetrabenazine has been considered to be effective as it depletes dopamine from nerve endings. This makes super-sensitivity reactions less likely in spite of an increase in receptor numbers. But the risk of depression is very high with tetrabenazine (similar to reserpine). Clonazepam, diazepam, vitamin E, and melatonin are other proposed management options.

Taylor et al., eds. *The Maudsley Prescribing Guidelines*, 8th edn. Taylor and Francis, 2005, p. 78.

50. B. Pimozide and thioridazine have been found to increase the QT interval. The QT interval (from the Q wave to the end of the T wave) varies with the heart rate, gender, and time of day. There are several different ways of correcting QT for heart rate (QTc), but the simplest method is using Bazett's formula. In this method, the corrected QT interval (QTc) is calculated by the equation $QTc = QT/\sqrt{RR}$. It is, however, uncertain whether QT_C has any greater clinical significance than the uncorrected QT interval. The normal QT interval is 340–430 ms, and irrespective of the heart rate, a QT interval >450 ms is probably risky. A prolonged QT interval can predispose to polymorphic ventricular arrhythmias (torsades de pointes).

Taylor et al., eds. *The Maudsley Prescribing Guidelines*, 8th edn. Taylor and Francis, 2005, p. 87.

51. C. Amoxapine is a TCA with fairly selective inhibition of noradrenaline reuptake. It also has D2 antagonist property. This pharmacological profile suggests a good option for the treatment of psychotic depression. But in addition to the side-effects of TCA, there is also an additional risk of side-effects associated with D2 antagonism.

Gelder MG et al., eds. *Shorter Oxford Textbook of Psychiatry*, 5th edn. Oxford University Press, 2006, p. 542.

52. C. Cardiovascular side-effects of tricyclics include hypotension and tachycardia. Conduction abnormalities, ECG changes, ventricular arrhythmias, and heart blocks are complications seen especially in people with pre-existing heart disease. Lofepramine is a tertiary amine which is metabolized to desipramine, a secondary amine. Inspite of being a tertiary amine, lofepramine is more selective for norepinephrine reuptake inhibition. It has a better side-effect profile compared to other TCAs. It is also less cardiotoxic than other TCAs.

Gelder MG et al., eds. *Shorter Oxford Textbook of Psychiatry*, 5th edn. Oxford University Press, 2006, p. 543.

53. C. SSRIs are safer than TCAs as far as cardiotoxicity, switch to mania, and seizures are concerned. But SSRIs are more prone to cause extrapyramidal reaction, possibly due to an increase in serotonin at 5HT heteroceptors on dopaminergic neurones. Some of the SSRIs may also have a low degree of intrinsic antagonistic action at the dopaminergic receptors.

Gelder MG et al., eds. *Shorter Oxford Textbook of Psychiatry*, 5th edn. Oxford University Press, 2006, p. 546.

54. E.   Serotonin syndrome is a potentially fatal syndrome occurring in the context of initiation or dose increase of a serotonergic agent. This syndrome is characterized by altered mental state, agitation, tremor, shivering, diarrhoea, hyper-reflexia, myoclonus, ataxia, and hyperthermia. It could also occur during combination antidepressant therapy. These include medications that exert their primary action through the serotonin receptor (SSRI, SNRI, buspirone, etc), MAOIs, and serotonin precursor tryptophan. Serotonin toxicity is also reported to occur when SSRIs are combined with medications whose mode of action is not known (lithium) or medications which may inhibit CYP enzymes and increase SSRI levels in plasma. Sternbach's criteria are used to diagnose serotonin syndrome.

Semple DM *et al.*, eds. *Oxford Handbook of Psychiatry*, 1st edn. Oxford University Press, 2005, p. 870.

55. B.   SSRIs are generally not sedating. Sometimes they can be activating, producing initial insomnia, anxiety, or panic attacks. They are relatively safer in overdose compared to TCAs. Apart from paroxetine and to some extent fluoxetine, most SSRIs have almost absent anticholinergic activity. SSRIs have been found to be more useful in obsessions than the other antidepressant groups.

Semple DM *et al.*, eds. *Oxford Handbook of Psychiatry*, 1st edn. Oxford University Press, 2005, p. 358.

56. B.   Incidence of hypertensive reaction is about 10% in patients who take MAOIs. Tyramine is a substance usually metabolized by MAO A in the intestinal mucosa. In patients who are taking MAOIs, the breakdown of tyramine is not adequate, leading to the 'cheese reaction'. Salbutamol, being an agonist at the adrenergic receptor, could precipitate a hypertensive crisis in patients taking MAOIs. The combination of TCAs and MAOIs could potentially induce severe postural hypotension. Side-effects of MAOIs include anticholinergic side-effects and insomnia, rather than sedation. Phenelzine, tranylcypromine, and isocarboxazid are irreversible inhibitors and non-selectively bind to both MAO A and MAO B. Moclobemide is a selective and reversible MAOI. Although the incidence is less, tyramine reaction can occur even with moclobemide.

Gelder MG *et al.*, eds. *Shorter Oxford Textbook of Psychiatry*, 5th edn. Oxford University Press, 2006, p. 551.

57. D.   Lithium is associated with leucocytosis and could be used therapeutically for carbamazepine- or clozapine-induced leucopenia. All the other drugs in the question are associated with leucopenia and agranulocytosis as a result of idiosyncratic drug reaction.

Taylor *et al.*, eds. *The Maudsley Prescribing Guidelines*, 8th edn. Taylor and Francis, 2005, p. 60.

58. E.   Lamotrigine acts by blocking voltage-gated sodium channels associated with glutamate receptors. Carbamazepine is an enzyme inducer and decreases lamotrigine levels. Valproate is an enzyme inhibitor and increases lamotrigine levels. So combining lamotrigine with carbamazepine or valproate requires caution. Lamotrigine has been found to be effective as a monotherapy for bipolar depression. It has not been found to be effective in acute mania or relapse prevention of mania in bipolar disorder. Lamotrigine does not induce CYP450 enzymes.

Semple DM *et al.*, eds. *Oxford Handbook of Psychiatry*, 1st edn. Oxford University Press, 2005, p. 320.

59. E. SIADH is an idiosyncratic reaction in response to treatment with antidepressants, especially SSRIs. Old age, diabetes, hypertension, impaired renal function, and chronic obstructive pulmonary disease (COPD) are risk factors for SIADH. SIADH usually presents as unexplained weakness and lethargy. In severe forms it can cause confusion and delirium. Serum Na^+ <125 mmol/l and a 24-h urine Na^+ >20 mmol/l or osmolality >100 mosml/kg are diagnostic indicators for SIADH. Withdrawal of the offending agent is the most effective intervention, apart from maintaining fluid balance. It is important to rule out other primary causes of SIADH before concluding it to be a drug-induced effect. It is known to occur with almost all classes of antidepressants.

Semple DM *et al.*, eds. *Oxford Handbook of Psychiatry*, 1st edn. Oxford University Press, 2005, p. 874.

60. B. Fluoxetine has a half-life of up to 72 hours. It also has an active metabolite with similar action, which prolongs the total duration of action up to 2 weeks (norfluoxetine). So, discontinuation reaction is less likely with fluoxetine. Paroxetine and citalopram have a half-life of 20 to 30 hours. Discontinuation reaction usually develops after at least a month of SSRI treatment and within 2–5 days after SSRI discontinuation or dose reduction. In general, gradual taper and stopping of the medications are indicated when SSRIs are used. Reinstatement of the same or a longer-acting SSRI can alleviate the symptoms, apart from using benzodiazepines. All classes of antidepressants are known to be associated with discontinuation reactions, including venlafaxine and amitriptyline.

Semple DM *et al.*, eds. *Oxford Handbook of Psychiatry*, 1st edn. Oxford University Press, 2005, p. 872.

1. **Which one of the following was a proponent of humane and moral treatment of insanity?**
   A. Anton Mesmer
   B. Phillipe Pinel
   C. Jacques Lacan
   D. Emil Krapelin
   E. Melanie Klein

2. **Morel was a French–Austrian physician associated with the term demence precoce. He is also associated with which of the following theories?**
   A. Regeneration theory
   B. Devolution theory
   C. Degeneration theory
   D. Segregation theory
   E. Integration theory

3. **Neurasthenia was originally described by which one of the following?**
   A. Beard
   B. Freud
   C. Jung
   D. Adler
   E. Engel

4. **Inducing malarial fever was proposed as a treatment for which of the following diseases?**
   A. Hysteria
   B. Neurasthenia
   C. Tourette's syndrome
   D. General paralysis of the insane
   E. Multiple sclerosis

5. **Which one of the following hormones was used to induce coma in the treatment of schizophrenia?**

   A. Thyroxine
   B. Cortisone
   C. Testosterone
   D. Insulin
   E. Parathormone

6. **Who among the following described hebephrenic schizophrenia?**

   A. Greisinger
   B. Falret and Baillarger
   C. Tuke
   D. Hecker
   E. Clouston

7. **Which one of the following terms was coined by Esquirol?**

   A. Nymphomania
   B. Monomania
   C. Hypomania
   D. Pseudomania
   E. Pyromania

8. **First-rank symptoms in schizophrenia were proposed by**

   A. Kurt Schneider
   B. Carl Schneider
   C. Manfred Bleuler
   D. Eugen Bleuler
   E. Emil Kraeplin

9. **All of the following are correctly matched EXCEPT**

   A. Ribot: anhedonia
   B. Sifneos: alexithymia
   C. Kahlbaum: cyclothymia
   D. Moreno: chorea
   E. Cameron: overinclusion

10. **The first antidepressants to be discovered were**

    A. SSRIs
    B. MAOIs
    C. TCAs
    D. Amphetamines
    E. Benzodiazepines

11. **Case studies have been traditionally useful in studying brain–behaviour relationships. In one of such case study Phineas Gage, a railway worker, sustained damage to which of the following brain areas?**
    A. Parietal lobe
    B. Hypothalamus
    C. Pineal gland
    D. Frontal lobe
    E. Temporal lobe

12. **Lithium was used in which of the following medical illnesses before being rediscovered for mania?**
    A. Gout
    B. Osteoarthritis
    C. Epilepsy
    D. Stroke
    E. Goitre

13. **Which one of the following is the oldest treatment method employed to cure mental illness?**
    A. Electroconvulsion
    B. Coma induction
    C. Trephination
    D. Lobotomy
    E. Rest cure

14. **Durkheim is a name associated with the study of which of the following phenomena?**
    A. Homicide
    B. Violence
    C. Truancy
    D. Arson
    E. Suicide

15. **Which of the following is a correct match with respect to diagnostic scales in psychiatry?**
    A. Negative symptoms: Jaspers
    B. Akathisia: Barnes
    C. Frontal battery: Folstein
    D. MMSE: Andreasen
    E. Formal thought disturbance: Hare

16. **Which one of the following is regarded as an illustrative case for classical conditioning in phobia?**

    A. Little Hans and horses
    B. Little Albert and rabbit
    C. Anna O
    D. Daniel Schreber
    E. Ratman

17 . **Who among the following used the term agoraphobia to describe a category of anxiety disorder?**

    A. Burton
    B. Schneider
    C. Westphal
    D. Jung
    E. Anna Freud

18. **Freud is regarded as the father of psychoanalysis. Which one of the following techniques was developed by Freud for his own clinical practice?**

    A. Narcoanalysis
    B. Polysomnography
    C. Free association
    D. Dissociation
    E. Mesmerism

19. **Phrenology refers to the study of which of the following concepts?**

    A. Study of free will
    B. Study of conscience
    C. Study of logic
    D. Study of skull contour
    E. Study of homunculus

20. **Schizophrenia was coined by Bleuler in 1911. The literal meaning of the term schizophrenia is**

    A. Split mind
    B. Split skull
    C. Fused mind
    D. Exploded will
    E. Split will

21. **Which of the following refers to the literal meaning of the term hysteria?**

    A. Wandering mind
    B. Wandering kidney
    C. Wandering uterus
    D. Wandering brain
    E. Wandering heart

22. **Which of the following diagnostic technique involved injecting air into subarachnoid space?**

    A. Myelography
    B. Pneumoencephalography
    C. Electroencephalography
    D. Encephalotomography
    E. Encephaloultrasonography

23. **In a large, multicentre trial reported in 1988, Kane demonstrated that clozapine was superior in treatment-resistant schizophrenia patients compared to which of the following drugs?**

    A. Haloperidol
    B. Chlorpromazine
    C. Olanzapine
    D. Fluphenazine
    E. Thoridazine

24. **Who is the proponent of primal therapy?**

    A. Arthur Janov
    B. Melanie Klein
    C. William Tuke
    D. Franz Alexander
    E. Mary Ainsworth

25. **Which of the following described delusions as un-understandable?**

    A. Jean Piaget
    B. Erik Erikson
    C. Karl Jaspers
    D. Eric Fromm
    E. Aaron Beck

26. **Choose the best explanation for the term spirituality:**

    A. Affiliation to a religious group
    B. Habitual practice of any religious activity
    C. Submission to existence of supreme powers, for example God
    D. Deeply held beliefs about the meaning of life
    E. Religious orientation without discrimination

27. **The International Pilot Study on Schizophrenia concluded that global, cultural, and social differences exist in which one of the following characters of schizophrenia?**

    A. Core symptoms
    B. Severity
    C. Outcome
    D. Dose of medications
    E. Gender distribution

28. **Which one of the following psychopathologies is influenced more significantly by cultural differences than the others listed?**

A. Delusions

B. Somatization

C. Hallucinations

D. Mania

E. Obsessions

29. **When using interpreters during psychiatric interview it is best NOT to**

A. Explain goals of the interview to the interpreter

B. Rotate different interpreters with the same patient

C. Provide debriefing to the interpreter after an emotional clinical encounter

D. Enquire about the interpreter's country of origin or social position

E. Encourage literal translation of the Mental State Examination

30. **Clinical samples of patients with anorexia nervosa show a trend towards which of the following social categories?**

A. Upper social class

B. Lower social class

C. Immigrant population

D. Poor literacy

E. More elderly parents

31. **Sick role includes all of the following EXCEPT**

A. Excuse from social responsibility

B. Expectation to seek help

C. Taking blame and responsibility for the illness

D. Perception of disease as undesirable

E. Attempts to restore previous state of health

32. **Which one of the following is NOT a component of high expressed emotions?**

A. Warmth

B. Over involvement

C. Critical comments

D. Enmeshment

E. Hostility

33. **High expressed emotions could be measured using which of the following instruments?**

A. Camberwell Assessment of Needs

B. Camberwell Family Interview

C. Simpson Angus Scale

D. Quality of Life Scale

E. Caregiver Burden Scale

34. **Effects of high expressed emotions could be mitigated to some extent in which one of the following situations?**

    A. The contact with family is less than 35 hours a week
    B. The family members are having mental health difficulties themselves
    C. The patient is married
    D. The patient has comorbid depression
    E. The patient has chronic rather than acute schizophrenia

35. **Association between crime and mental illness is difficult to study. This is due to which of the following reasons?**

    A. Most criminals are mentally ill
    B. Criminals are deceptive about mental illness
    C. Crime is over reported
    D. Captives are not representative of all criminals
    E. Mental illness is rarely independent of the crime committed

36. **Stigma associated with mental illness could potentially be reduced by all of the following interventions EXCEPT**

    A. Destigmatization campaigns
    B. Increasing community living of severely mentally ill people
    C. Educating the public about mental illness
    D. Legislation against social discrimination
    E. Improving broadcasting standards

37. **Which of the following is NOT true with respect to stigma against mental illness?**

    A. Stigma leads to social exclusion
    B. Stigma can prolong the duration of depression in a patient
    C. Stigma is seen even against mentally ill professionals
    D. Stigma has reduced substantially in the last two decades
    E. Stigma perceived by patients varies with their diagnosis

38. **The term acculturation refers to which of the following?**

    A. Adoption of beliefs and values of one cultural group by another
    B. Migration of civilizations in need of food and shelter
    C. Adoption of civilized social norms by a culturally weaker group
    D. Acceptance of rules and regulations of a mental health institute
    E. The tendency for a cultural group to enforce their values on another group

39. **Koro is an anxiety state seen most commonly in which of the following geographical zone?**

    A. Latin America
    B. South-east Asia
    C. India
    D. Alaskan natives
    E. Siberia

40. Which one of the following is a culture-bound syndrome characterized by an exaggerated startle reaction in middle-aged women?

A. Piblokto

B. Latah

C. Brain fag

D. Windigo

E. Susto

41. In the UK, the annual prevalence of hallucinations is higher in which of the following racial groups?

A. Asians

B. Caribbeans

C. Americans

D. Whites

E. Australian Jews

42. Which of the following is true regarding increased incidence of schizophrenia among migrant population?

A. It depends on the country of origin

B. It could be explained by drug use

C. It is due to genetic factors

D. It is generation limited

E. It is strongly related to lower socioeconomic status

43. Which of the following theories holds that mental illness is a result of societal influence?

A. Causation theory

B. Drift theory

C. Labelling theory

D. Social disintegration theory

E. Social agent theory

44. A patient with learning disability cannot understand the implications of hospitalization. But he does not resist being admitted to a hospital. Which of the following best describes his mental capacity status?

A. Compliant and capable

B. Compliant but not capable

C. Non-compliant and incapable

D. Non-compliant but capable

E. None of the above

45. **A patient decides to be on the waiting list for 12 months untill she could see a psychotherapist. Choose an ethical principle relevant to this scenario:**

   A. Confidentiality
   B. Distributive justice
   C. Therapeutic privilege
   D. Non-maleficience
   E. Autonomy

46. **A test for capacity to make treatment decisions includes all of the following EXCEPT**

   A. Ability to understand the choice
   B. Belief in the information given
   C. Ability to analyse benefits and harm
   D. Ability to retain information long enough to analyse them
   E. Ability to communicate a decision

47. **Which is the most important ethical principle underlying informed consent?**

   A. Beneficience
   B. Autonomy
   C. Non-maleficience
   D. Justice
   E. Paternalism

48. **Over-riding patient confidentiality cannot be substantiated reasonably if it is carried out under which of the following situations?**

   A. Grave danger to a third party
   B. Disclosure of information is required by law
   C. Child protection involved
   D. Under court order
   E. Following the Death of the patient

49. **Which of the following cannot be considered as an exception to direct informed consent?**

   A. Waiver
   B. Detention under mental health act
   C. Emergencies where full information cannot be given
   D. Incompetent patient
   E. Passively compliant patient

50. **In ethology, imprinting refers to which of the following processes?**

   A. Learning modified by consequences
   B. Learning independent of developmental age
   C. Slow learning of parental behaviours
   D. Learning neonatal reflexes in human beings
   E. None of the above

51. **If a patient reveals murderous intentions against his wife, a psychiatrist is duty bound to inform both police and the wife. This principle is derived from which of the following medicolegal illustrations?**
    A. Tarasoff's case
    B. Bournewood case
    C. McNaughten's case
    D. Gillick's case
    E. Shipman's case

52. **Which of the following best describes the difference between the terms handicap and impairment?**
    A. Handicap refers to loss of social role
    B. Impairment refers to loss of social role
    C. Handicap refers to a structural defect
    D. Impairment refers to inability to perform a complex task
    E. Handicap refers to irreversible loss

53. **Fathers of schizophrenia patients originate from higher social class than the patients themselves. This exemplifies which of the following theories?**
    A. Social causation
    B. Social disintegration
    C. Social drift
    D. Social labelling
    E. Social construction

54. **The Helsinki declaration is applicable in which of the following scenarios?**
    A. A 24-year-old man is comatose and needs blood transfusion
    B. A 13-year-old girl asks for contraception
    C. A Jehovah's witness refuses blood transfusion for his 5-year-old child
    D. A 34-year-old man volunteers for a neuroimaging study
    E. A 94-year-old lady refuses to move to a nursing home

55. **Which one of the following occupations carries a high risk of eating disorders?**
    A. Modelling
    B. Law
    C. Nursing
    D. Marketing
    E. Teaching

56. **Under the principle of common law which of the following can be done without a patient's consent?**

    A. Blood sample can be drawn after paracetamol overdose in an emergency
    B. Liver transplantation can be done on a suicidal patient
    C. A psychiatric inpatient can be detained overnight if they attempt to leave
    D. Contraceptives can be implanted to a young lady with mania
    E. Depot antipsychotics could be given for agitation

57. **'Run amok' involves sudden dissociative reaction which can lead to multiple homicide or suicide. It is best classified under which of the following categories?**

    A. Dissociation reaction
    B. Somatoform disorders
    C. Culture-bound syndrome
    D. Substance use disorder
    E. Delusional disorder

58. **Who first used the word 'psychiatry' (or 'psychiatrie') to describe the profession?**

    A. Reil
    B. Rush
    C. Deniker
    D. Kline
    E. Charcot

59. **One of the following is a major proponent of the antipsychiatry movement?**

    A. William Osler
    B. Thomas Szasz
    C. Aubrey Lewis
    D. Henry Maudsley
    E. Adolf Meyer

60. **Which of the following is NOT routinely considered as boundary violations in a therapeutic relationship?**

    A. Touching except handshake
    B. Treating friends or relatives
    C. Personal disclosure
    D. Interpretation of emotionally neutral statements
    E. Colluding with a patient against a third party

1. B.   Phillipe Pinel (1745–1826) was working at Salpetriere in Paris at the time of the French Revolution. He insisted on releasing patients from chains in asylums, emphasized systematic clinical observations using case records and championed humane treatment of the mentally ill. Anton Mesmer was a proponent of mesmerism, a form of clinical suggestion. Jacques Lacan is known as the 'French Freud'. Melanie Klein was an object relations theorist.

Gelder MG et al., eds. New Oxford Textbook of Psychiatry. Oxford University Press, 2000, p. 17.

2. C.   Degeneration theory maintained that most forms of insanity resulted from continuous deterioration of mental faculties. More alarmingly, it also stated that hereditary transmission of nervous dysfunction was produced by noxious environmental factors. Morel was the proponent of degeneration theory.

Gelder MG et al., eds. New Oxford Textbook of Psychiatry. Oxford University Press, 2000, p.19.

3. A.   American neurologist, Beard, described neurasthenia in 1880. This is retained in the ICD-10, and is the closest diagnosis to the present day chronic fatigue syndrome. Various terms, including myalgic encephalomyelitis and viral fatigue syndrome, are in vogue in an attempt to emphasize infectious/ inflammatory origin of this illness.

Gelder MG et al., eds. New Oxford Textbook of Psychiatry. Oxford University Press, 2000, p. 21.

4. D.   General paresis or paralysis of the insane (GPI, also called as paralytic dementia) is a rare encephalitic illness. GPI was common in the past due to syphilis. Malaria therapy for GPI was proposed by Wagner von Jauregg, a Nobel laureate. Manic presentation was common in GPI. GPI has almost disappeared now, though with the rising HIV pandemic it is speculated to have resurgence in the future.

Gelder MG et al., eds. New Oxford Textbook of Psychiatry. Oxford University Press, 2000, p. 21.

5. D.   Insulin coma therapy for severe mental illness was introduced by Sakel in 1933. This was a potentially fatal treatment complicated by seizures and encephalopathy. Chemically induced seizures were also employed around the same period (von Meduna) for treating schizophrenia.

Gelder MG et al., eds. New Oxford Textbook of Psychiatry. Oxford University Press, 2000, p. 21.

6. D.   Hecker described hebephrenia – characterized by adolescent onset with disorganized behaviour and incongruent affect. Hecker was a pupil of Karl Kahlbaum, and some consider that he only popularized the notion of hebephrenic schizophrenia, which was originally proposed by Kahlbaum. Sir Thomas Clouston is associated with 'developmental insanity'. William Tuke opened the Retreat in York, promoting moral treatment and unchaining the insane. Falret and Baillarger are associated with folie circulaire (manic depression) while Greisinger developed views on tha neuropathological basis for psychiatric disorders.

Johnstone EC et al., eds. Companion to Psychiatric Studies, 7th edn. Churchill Livingstone, 2004, p. 3.

7. B. Monomania was described by Esquirol and it is similar to the present day concept of delusional disorder. Nymphomania was coined in 1775, by a French doctor Bienville, from Greek *nymphe* meaning 'bride'. It was used to describe excessive sexual desire seen in some women. The term hypomania was coined by Mendel (1881).

Bynum B. Monomania. *Lancet* 2003; **362**: 1425.

Angst J, *et al.* Toward a re-definition of subthreshold bipolarity: epidemiology and proposed criteria for bipolar-II, minor bipolar disorders and hypomania. *Journal of Affective Disorders* 2003; **73**, 133–146.

8. A. Kurt Schneider proposed first-rank symptoms – neither diagnostic nor prognostic but only indicative of schizophrenia. Eugen Bleuler used the term schizophrenia in 1911. Carl Schneider classified many forms of formal thought disturbances; later he was closely associated with the Nazi movement in Germany, promoting 'euthanasia' for mentally retarded and epileptic patients.

Gelder MG *et al.*, eds. *New Oxford Textbook of Psychiatry*. Oxford University Press, 2000, p. 568.

9. D. Moreno described psychodrama, not chorea. He also introduced sociometry. Anhedonia stands for inability to obtain pleasure from activities; alexithymia is a difficulty in verbalizing emotional states; Cyclothymia, retained in ICD-10, is a minor subsyndromal form of bipolar illness described by Kahlbaum; Cameron described overinclusion as a part of formal thought disturbances.

Gelder MG *et al.*, eds. *New Oxford Textbook of Psychiatry*. Oxford University Press, 2000, p. 1446.

10. B. Monoamine oxidase inhibitors were the earliest antidepressants. They were serendipitously discovered when iproniazid, an antitubercular antibiotic, was found to have mood-lifting properties. This was reported by Bloch in 1954.

Gelder MG *et al.*, eds. *New Oxford Textbook of Psychiatry*. Oxford University Press, 2000, p. 1293.

11. D. Phineas Gage was a railway workman whose frontal lobe (especially the ventromedial prefrontal area) was accidentally drilled out by an iron bar. He survived the terrible accident but had significant personality and behavioural change, stimulating interest in studying functions of the frontal lobe.

Johnstone EC *et al.*, eds. *Companion to Psychiatric Studies*, 7th edn. Churchill Livingstone, 2004, p. 133.

12. A. Lithium was brought to the attention of psychiatric practice in 1949 by Australian, John Cade, who highlighted its mood-stabilizing effect. Lithium water was a popular 'tonic for aches and pains' and was used for gout before this discovery.

Johnstone EC *et al.*, eds. *Companion to Psychiatric Studies*, 7th edn. Churchill Livingstone, 2004, p. 256.

13. C. Trephination refers to drilling holes in skulls to release evil spirit that were believed to haunt the insane. This practice is noted even in prehistoric skulls dated 6500 BC. Electroconvulsion was introduced by Cerletti and Bini in the early part of the twentieth century, while Moniz proposed neurosurgical methods to treat psychiatric disorders.

Rutkow IM. Moments in surgical history – trephination: how did they do it? *Archives of Surgery* 2000; **135**: 1119.

14. E.   Durkheim described anomic, altruistic, and egoistic suicide. In anomie, the patient feels let down by society and fails to follow norms. In altruistic suicide, over involvement with a particular social group leads to significant alteration in one's self identity and the suicide is for the group cause rather than personal cause, for example hara-kiri of a soldier. Egoistic suicide refers to those suicides in people who are not strongly integrated into any social group, for example lack of family integration in unmarried persons.

Sadock BJ and Sadock VA. *Kaplan & Sadock's Synopsis of Psychiatry: Behavioral Sciences/Clinical Psychiatry*, 10th edn. Lippincott Williams & Wilkins, 2007, p. 900.

15. B.   Barnes' Akathisia Rating Scale is used to measure akathisia, a side-effect of antipsychotics characterized by both subjective and, later, objective restlessness. Folstein described MMSE in a seminal paper; Andreasen devised the Thought Language and Communication scale to measure formal thought disturbance; Kay's PANSS (positive and negative symptom scale) can measure negative symptoms; Hare is a name associated with a psychopathy checklist used by forensic services.

Barnes TRE. The Barnes akathisia rating scale – revisited. *Journal of Psychopharmacology* 2003; **17**: 365–370.

16. B.   Little Albert learnt to avoid rabbits after a loud noise induced fear in him whenever he played with a white rat. This fear later generalized to white rabbits (Watson and Rayner 1920). Anna O was a patient with 'hysteria' treated by Freud and Breuer. Ratman was also a patient of Freud who had OCD, while Schreber had delusional disorder.

Sadock BJ and Sadock VA. *Kaplan & Sadock's Synopsis of Psychiatry: Behavioral Sciences/Clinical Psychiatry*, 10th edn. Lippincott Williams & Wilkins, 2007, p. 142.
Watson JB, Rayner R. Conditioned emotional reactions. *Journal of Experimental Psychology* 1920; **3**: 1–14.

17. C.   Robert Burton wrote 'The Anatomy of Melancholy' in which some description of symptoms suggestive of agoraphobia is seen together with the account of depressive illness. In 1871, Carl Otto Westphal coined the term agoraphobia to describe several of his patients who experienced severe anxiety when walking through streets or open squares. Schneider proposed first-rank symptoms; Jung belonged to the psychoanalytic school. Anna Freud, Freud's daughter, was involved in classifying defence mechanisms and also in child psychoanalysis.

Callard F. 'The sensation of infinite vastness'; or, the emergence of agoraphobia in the late 19th century *Environment and Planning: Society and Space* 2006; **24**: 873–889.

18. C.   Free association was a popular technique used by Freudian analysts. Having learnt hypnosis from Charcot, neurologist-turned-psychoanalyst Freud developed the method of free association in which patients were encouraged to speak about their thoughts without distraction or censure. This was intended to be a therapeutic method, though later adapted largely as an interview technique. Narcoanalysis involves using barbiturates as truth serum. Dissociation is a psychological mechanism and not a clinical technique. Mesmerism or animal magnetism was developed by Anton Mesmer.

Johnstone EC et al., eds. *Companion to Psychiatric Studies*, 7th edn. Churchill Livingstone, 2004, p. 5.

19. D.   Phrenology was a popular theory which claimed to determine personality and diagnose/predict mental symptoms using the shape of the skull. It was developed by the German physician Gall and was very popular in the mid 1800s. Phrenologists used their bare hands and palms to feel for fissures or dents in their patients' skulls. With this information, the phrenologist would report on the character of the patient; its popularity reached extremes when marriages and recruitment were advised by phrenologists.

Simpson D. Phrenology and the neurosciences: contributions of F. J. Gall and J. G. Spurzheim. *Australia and New Zealand Journal of Surgery* 2005; **75**: 475.

20.A.   The term 'schizophrenia' stands for split personality. Even today this is confused with more dramatic multiple personality disorder by some of the lay public. The term was coined by Eugene Bleuler in 1911. It is derived from the Greek words 'schizo' (split) and 'phrene' (mind). Bleuler intended to use the name in order to capture the functional dissociation between personality, thinking, memory, and perception in a patient with schizophrenia.

Gelder MG et al., eds. New Oxford Textbook of Psychiatry. Oxford University Press, 2000, p. 568.

21. C.   The term hysteria stands for 'wandering uterus'. It was incorrectly observed that hysteria affects only women. The uterus is a major morphological difference between a man and a woman; hence, rather simplistically, it was believed that uterus was the site of problems in hysteria. Also it was believed that unmarried women often had this wandering uterus that could be tied down by wedlock, leading to a reduction in hysterical symptoms following marriage. It was even believed in a Greek myth that this wandering uterus could strangulate a person, leading to hysterical globus or aphonia! Unusual treatments, including pelvic massage to induce orgasm, were offered to cure hysteria later in history.

Sadock BJ and Sadock VA. Kaplan & Sadock's Synopsis of Psychiatry: Behavioral Sciences/Clinical Psychiatry, 10th edn. Lippincott Williams & Wilkins, 2007, p. 634.

22. B.   Dandy, in 1919, used pneumoencephalogram as a diagnostic technique to visualize the brain. This technique showed enlarged ventricles in patients with schizophrenia, which was later confirmed by investigations using various other imaging modalities that developed later. There was a high fatality rate associated with pneumoencephalogram.

Semrad EV and Finley KH. A note on the pneumoencephalogram and electroencephalogram findings in chronic mental patients. Psychiatric Quarterly 1963; **17**: 76–80.

23. B.   Kane revived the use of clozapine through his milestone study. He compared chlorpromazine and clozapine in a treatment-resistant sample and demonstrated clozapine's superiority in this instance (in 1988) leading to FDA approval (in 1989). The multicentre trial showed that 30% of clozapine-treated patients will respond in 6 weeks while 60% will respond in 6 months. On the other hand, only 4% improved on chlorpromazine in combination with benztropine.

Johnstone EC et al., eds. Companion to Psychiatric Studies, 7th edn. Churchill Livingstone, 2004, p. 262.

24.A.   Primal therapy refers to a trauma-focused treatment proposed by Arthur Janov. Primal therapy claims that only through direct experience of pain and emotions, could any psychological treatment work. Other talking therapies use higher cortical cognitive processes to talk about emotional experience while primal therapy attempts to engage lower brain centres during psychotherapy.

Janov A. Towards a new consciousness. Journal of Psychosomatic Research 1977; **21**: 333–339.

25. C.   Jaspers was both a psychiatrist and a philosopher. He studied psychopathology in depth; the descriptive psychopathology and psychiatric phenomenology used in current psychiatric practice are largely Jasper's contributions. According to him, a specific quality of delusions is their 'un-understandability'. This distinguished primary delusions from delusion-like ideas or secondary delusions that arose out of a different psychopathology, for example hallucinations.

Jones H et al. Jaspers was right after all – delusions are distinct from normal beliefs. British Journal of Psychiatry 2003; **183**: 285–286.
see also
Owen G et al. Jaspers' concept of primary delusion. British Journal of Psychiatry 2004; **185**: 77–78.

26. D. Contrary to widely held belief, spirituality is not defined as affiliation to religious practice or accepting God. It rather refers to deeply held beliefs about the meaning of one's life.

Kay J and Tasman A, eds. *Essentials of Psychiatry.* Wiley, 2006, p. 23.

27. C. The IPSS (International Pilot Study on Schizophrenia) was a global, multicentre study carried out by the WHO. The main finding was a strikingly similar core symptom profile irrespective of cultural differences and more or less similar life-time morbid risk (though this has been disputed; See McGrath NAPE lecture 2004). Surprisingly, outcome of schizophrenia was better in the developing, rather than the developed countries.

McGrath JJ. The surprisingly rich contours of schizophrenia epidemiology. *Archives of General Psychiatry* 2007; **64**: 14–16.

McGrath JJ. Myths and plain truths about schizophrenia epidemiology – the NAPE lecture 2004. *Acta Psychiatrica Scandinavica* 2005; **111**: 4–11.

28. B. Somatization is consistently found to be higher among South Asian populations, especially in females. Linguistic differences could explain an apparent inability to verbalize emotions, leading to requests for medical interventions for physical symptoms. Cultural sensitivity is essential to detect undiagnosed depression in different ethnic groups.

Bhui K and Hotopf M. Somatization disorder. *British Journal of Hospital Medicine* 1997; **58**: 145–149.

29. B. Using different interpreters for different sessions of clinical encounter with the same patient will lead to confusion and needless anxiety due to the presence of a new person during each doctor–patient meeting. It is advisable to stick to the same interpreter when dealing with a particular patient. Knowing the interpreter's social and ethnic background might help in utilizing the interpretation better. Also, the Mental State Examination can be misinterpreted by a lay person – it is often necessary to instruct the interpreter to translate certain parts of the clinical interview verbatim.

Kay J and Tasman A, eds. *Essentials of Psychiatry.* Wiley, 2006, p. 27.

30. A. An unequal distribution of social class is noted in anorexia. Higher representation from upper classes of society, good literacy rates, and higher frequency of non-immigrant populations is noted among clinical samples of anorexia patients. This strengthens the aspect of culture specificity of anorexia nervosa.

Gelder MG *et al.*, eds. *New Oxford Textbook of Psychiatry.* Oxford University Press, 2000, p. 836

31. C. Sick role, as defined by Parsons, excludes patient from taking all responsibility for becoming ill. It is perceived that illness is unavoidable and any ill person must seek help, as illness is undesirable and an attempt must be made to restore the previous state of health. Untill this happens the person is relieved of certain social responsibilities. This social perception of illness drives a person to occupy what is collectively termed as the sick role.

Kay and Tasman A, eds. *Essentials of Psychiatry.* Wiley, 2006, p. 679.

32. D. Enmeshment has not been discussed as a component of expressed emotions (EE). Enmeshment stands for deranged family dynamics, characterized by blurring of normal hierarchy and intergenerational boundaries in a family. Enmeshment is linked to various child psychiatry problems, including eating disorders. EE is characterized by warmth, hostility, and critical comments and emotional over-involvement. High EE is implicated in relapse of various psychiatric illnesses, especially schizophrenia. It is also demonstrated that being on long-term antipsychotics can alleviate the relapse-provoking effect of a high EE environment to some extent. Vaughn and Leff studied EE in depth.

Gelder MG *et al.*, eds. *New Oxford Textbook of Psychiatry.* Oxford University Press, 2000, p. 603.

Leff J and Vaughn C. *Expressed Emotion in Families.* New York: Guilford Press, 1985.

33. B. The Camberwell Assessment of Needs scale, also called as CAN, was developed by the Section of Community Psychiatry (PRiSM) at the Institute of Psychiatry. It is a tool for assessing the needs of people with severe and enduring mental illness, including both health and social needs. It has clinical and research versions, and also a shorter version for routine use. The Camberwell Family Interview is a different scale from CAN, and assesses the feelings and experiences of relatives with regard to a patient's admission to hospital. In the Camberwell Family Interview, three measures of EE – criticism, hostility, and emotional over-involvement – are assessed.

Leff J and Vaughn C. *Expressed Emotion in Families.* Guilford Press, New York, 1985.

34. A. It has been shown that the effect of high expressed emotions on relapse of psychotic episodes is lesser if contact with family members lasts less than 35 hours a week. This dose–response relationship adds strength to the role of the family's emotional expression on the course of schizophrenia. The degree of EE can be higher if any of the family members has mental health difficulties themselves.

Johnstone EC et al., eds. *Companion to Psychiatric Studies,* 7th edn. Churchill Livingstone, 2004, p. 404.

35. D. It is widely acknowledged that captives may not be the ideal, representative sample of everyone who indulges in criminal activity. Captives may be a special population with lower than normal skills to escape or avoid a sentence or arrest. Often the IQ of captured criminals may be lower than the IQ of non-captured criminals, on average. So studying captives for the rate of mental illness or effect on crime secondary to treating mental illness could not be generalized to wider social criminalities. Most criminals are mentally sound. Crime is under-reported rather over reported, on the whole.

Johnstone EC et al., eds. *Companion to Psychiatric Studies,* 7th edn. Churchill Livingstone, 2004, p. 703.

36. B. Various measures to combat stigma has shown only modest benefits over the century. Destigmatization campaigns, public education, and vigilant media policy can be helpful. It is clear that in the past few decades, the closure of asylums and psychiatric hospitals has increased community living of patients with mental health problems. But this has not translated into lower rates of stigma and discrimination – if anything this has got worse, assuming different forms.

Byrne P. Stigma of mental illness and ways of diminishing it. *Advances in Psychiatric Treatment* 2000; **6**: 65–72.

37. D. Stigma has not reduced in anyway over last two decades in spite of improved literacy rates. The perceived stigma is more generic for mental illness and does vary with the diagnosis to some extent. Stigma leads to delayed help seeking and social exclusion, making outcome worse.

Byrne P. Stigma of mental illness and ways of diminishing it. *Advances in Psychiatric Treatment* 2000; **6**: 65–72.

38. A. Acculturation is a social–anthropological phenomenon which refers to the adoption of cultural practices of one group by another due to the effect of living close to each other. It does not refer to being civilized or non-civilized in cultural practice. The tendency for a cultural group to enforce their values on another group is called assimilation. Acceptance of rules and regulations of a mental health institute is related to the process of institutionalization, described by Goffman.

Sadock BJ and Sadock VA. *Kaplan & Sadock's Synopsis of Psychiatry: Behavioral Sciences/Clinical Psychiatry,* 10th edn. Lippincott Williams & Wilkins, 2007, p. 168.
Goffman E. *Asylums. Essays on the social situation of mental patients and other inmates.* Harmondsworth: Penguin, 1961.

39. B. Koro is a culture-bound syndrome that is most often seen as genital retraction anxiety rather than delusional state. It usually affects young males, and is accompanied by anxiety that genitals are shrinking. It is an acute condition with favourable prognosis compared to chronic psychotic illnesses. It is often reported in Malaysia, Taiwan, Philippines, and other parts of south-east Asia. It is referred to as Shook Yang in Japan. Koro literally means head of a turtle (which retracts).

Gelder MG *et al.*, eds. *New Oxford Textbook of Psychiatry*. Oxford University Press, 2000, p. 1062.

40. B. Latah is a culture-bound syndrome seen mainly in women in south-east Asia. It is characterized by severe startle response together with loss of control over behaviour, echolalia, and echopraxia. Such patients are noted to obey any commands issued to them.

Gelder MG *et al.*, eds. *New Oxford Textbook of Psychiatry*. Oxford University Press, 2000, p. 1063.

41. B. The prevalence of 'all cause' hallucinations are higher in the Caribbean population living in the UK compared to other ethnic groups. It is noted to be 2.5 times more common in this group. South Asian migrants come next in the list, followed by native White populations. Cultural differences exist not only in disease prevalence but also in non-clinical but abnormal mental experiences measured in community samples.

Johns LC, Nazroo JY, *et al.* Occurrence of hallucinatory experiences in a community sample and ethnic variations. *British Journal of Psychiatry* 2002; **180**: 174–178.

42. E. It is now accepted that immigration is a clear risk factor for developing schizophrenia, irrespective of the prevalence rates in the country of origin, genetic loading, or cannabis use. This effect is not limited to the generation that migrates – it extends to the second generation immigrants as demonstrated in the AESOP Study in the UK. It has also been shown that in neighbourhoods where minority status is significant due to the high population of majority ethnic group in the locality and poor socioeconomic status of immigrants, incidence of schizophrenia is increased. This applies to any minority group irrespective of racial status.

Cooper B. Immigration and schizophrenia: The social causation hypothesis revisited. *British Journal of Psychiatry* 2005; **186**: 361–363.

43. C. Labelling theory was applied to explain mental illness in 1966 by Thomas Scheff. He claimed that mental illness is manifested solely as a result of societal influence. The society views certain actions as deviant. A label of mental illness is placed on those who exhibit deviant behaviours in order to explain these behaviours. The expectations then placed on these individuals unconsciously change their behaviour – giving them the role of mentally ill. Social causation and drift theories attempt to explain the association between lower socioeconomic status and mental illness. Social causation theory proposes that low socioeconomic status breeds mental illnesses. Social drift theory takes the view that a decline in social status occurs following development of mental illnesses.

Johnstone EC *et al.*, eds. *Companion to Psychiatric Studies*, 7th edn. Churchill Livingstone, 2004, p. 123.

44. B. Often patients who lack capacity to make treatment decisions agree to follow a treatment plan passively. This special group is termed 'compliant not capable'. Learning disability services, dementia care, and geriatric care often face challenge with such patients. The Bournewood case refers to a patient with autism who was kept in hospital against the wishes of his carers as he complied with hospital admission. Though he did not have capacity to decide on his treatment he was not detained under the mental health act as he was compliant to stay at the hospital. This case revealed a wide gap in English mental health law.

Gelder MG *et al.*, eds. *New Oxford Textbook of Psychiatry*. Oxford University Press, 2000, p. 36.

45. B. Justice is one of four primary ethical principles. Justice is the moral obligation to act on the basis of fair judgement between competing claims. Justice is classified into: (1) fair distribution of scarce resources (distributive justice); (2) respect for people's rights (rights based justice); and (3) respect for morally acceptable laws (legal justice). In health ethics, distributive justice means equity for all where 'equals are equally treated'; it concerns economic distribution and health-care resource allocation.

Gillon R. Medical ethics: four principles plus attention to scope. *British Medical Journal* 1994; **309**: 184–8.

46. B. Capacity by definition is a legal concept; it refers to the ability to enter into valid contracts. Every adult is presumed to have capacity unless proved otherwise. Capacity is also task specific; one can have capacity to decide on treatment but can lack capacity to dispose of an estate. A test for capacity includes: (1) able to understand the nature of a decision that needs to be made; (2) able to weigh risks and benefits of any decision; (3) able to retain information long enough to make a decision; and (4) able to communicate the decision clearly. It is not necessary for the patient to believe in the information given to him.

Johnstone EC *et al.*, eds. *Companion to Psychiatric Studies*, 7th edn. Churchill Livingstone, 2004, p. 736.

47. B. For an informed consent to be valid, as a general rule, five areas of information must be provided: (1) description of the medical condition or problem; (2) nature and purpose of the proposed treatment; (3) risks and benefits of the proposed treatment; (4) viable alternatives to the proposed treatment; and (5) prognosis with and without treatment. The most important ethical principle preserved by obtaining informed consent is that of patient autonomy.

Sadock BJ and Sadock VA. *Kaplan & Sadock's Synopsis of Psychiatry: Behavioral Sciences/Clinical Psychiatry*, 10th edn. Lippincott Williams & Wilkins, 2007, p. 1372.

48. E. Personal information should not be disclosed to a third party without the patient's express consent, except when: (1) serious risk to third parties outweighs the interests on patient's privacy, for example child abuse; (2) disclosure of information is required by law, for example a notifiable disease; and (3) patient explicitly agrees to disclosure to a third party. Death of a patient does not waive one's responsibility to maintain confidentiality.

Sadock BJ and Sadock VA. *Kaplan & Sadock's Synopsis of Psychiatry: Behavioral Sciences/Clinical Psychiatry*, 10th edn. Lippincott Williams & Wilkins, 2007, p. 1387.

49. E. When a person is passively compliant it is necessary to consider absence of informed consent. This is often seen when patients are prescribed ECT – without knowing all required information, they will agree for a course of treatment passively as the doctor has prescribed it. Legal privilege is the right to maintain secrecy or confidentiality when summoned by court. The right of legal privilege belongs to the patient. Therapeutic privilege is different from this legal privilege. Therapeutic privilege is used when a psychiatrist withholds information in the belief that giving a patient all of the information would harm the patient. This is not commonly practised. While detaining a patient under the mental health act, often there is no consent from the patient for hospitalization. But this is commonly done against patient's approval on the grounds of safety of the patient and the others. An incompetent person is one who is incapable of giving informed consent; in which case, consent can be granted only by that person's guardian, or other persons with legal authority to give consent (e.g. a lasting power of attorney for health-care issues). Consent is presumed when a person is suffering from an emergent situation that requires treatment but is unable to give consent. Waiver is a situation where a patient asks the therapist not to give him a particular part of health information as that would be detrimental for him to know it. Again, this is rarely used.

Kay J and Tasman A, eds. *Essentials of Psychiatry*. Wiley, 2006, p. 88.

50. E. Ethology refers to the biological study of animal behaviour. Imprinting is a specialized form of learning which occurs early in life (critical phase). The exposure to the stimulus situation must occur during the critical period, and the exposure can be of short duration without any reinforcement. This type of learning is particularly resistant to change. It has not been clearly demonstrated in human infants so far.

Sadock BJ and Sadock VA. *Kaplan & Sadock's Synopsis of Psychiatry: Behavioral Sciences/Clinical Psychiatry*, 10th edn. Lippincott Williams & Wilkins, 2007, p. 160.

51. A. Two months before killing his exgirlfriend Tarasoff, Poddar had declared his intentions to his psychotherapist. The psychotherapist tried to have Poddar detained but he was soon released. Police were informed of the risk, but the court ruled that apart from a duty of care to the patient, and duty to protect by informing the police, there is a duty to warn the third party directly. This is called the Tarasoff ruling.

Sadock BJ and Sadock VA. *Kaplan & Sadock's Synopsis of Psychiatry: Behavioral Sciences/Clinical Psychiatry*, 10th edn. Lippincott Williams & Wilkins, 2007, p. 1374.

52. A. Impairment (I) is defined as any loss or abnormality of a bodily structure or function. Disability (D) is the restriction to perform an activity in a normal manner due to the impairment. The social disadvantage for a given individual in terms of role fulfilment resulting from the disability is called handicap (H) (I leads to D; D leads to H). Reversibility of loss is not considered as a discriminating feature in defining handicap.

Semple DM *et al.*, eds. *Oxford Handbook of Psychiatry*, 1st edn. Oxford University Press, 2005, p. 688.

53. C. Goldberg conducted a survey of a national sample of males aged 25–34 on their first admission to a mental hospital in England and Wales for schizophrenia. This showed an expected excess of patients in lower social class v Lower economic class was seen as a cause for schizophrenia (social causation). But when the social class distribution of the fathers at the time of the patients' birth was studied, it transpired to be very similar to that of the general population. This is explained by the hypothesis that schizophrenia results in a downward drift of socioeconomic status rather than poverty being a cause for schizophrenia. (This social drift hypothesis was first suggested by the Chicago study of Faris and Dunham, 1922–1934).

Goldberg EM and Morrison SL. Schizophrenia and social class. *British Journal of Psychiatry* 1963; **109**: 785–802.

54. D. The Helsinki declaration is associated with research ethics. The efforts to streamline ethical principles of conducting research on human subjects started following the Second World War. Gillick competence refers to the assessment of ability of a child (16 years or younger) to consent to his or her own medical treatment, without the need for parental permission.

Goodyear MDE, *et al.* The Declaration of Helsinki. *British Medical Journal* 2007; **335**: 624–625.

55. A. Ballet dancers and models have a high prevalence of anorexia nervosa as a result of pressures to sustain a slim figure consistent with their professional requirements.

Gelder MG *et al.*, eds. *New Oxford Textbook of Psychiatry*. Oxford University Press, 2000, p. 836.

56. A. Common law principle of necessity allows medical interventions only if they are life saving, emergency measures. Irreversible procedures such as transplantation cannot be carried out. It is not good practice to administer depot under 'emergency' situations. Psychiatric detention must follow Mental Health Act principles whenever required.

Hewson B. The law on managing patients who harm themselves and deliberately refuse treatment. *British Medical Journal* 1999; **319**: 905–907.

57. C. Running amok (derived from Malay word *amuk*, meaning 'mad with anger') is a Malaysian culture bound syndrome. It usually affects a young male who will develop a sudden frenzy and acquire a weapon in an attempt to kill or injure anyone indiscriminately. Amok episodes can lead to serious violence or suicide.

Gelder MG *et al.*, eds. *New Oxford Textbook of Psychiatry*. Oxford University Press, 2000, p. 1063.

58. A. Johann Christian Reil coined the term psychiatry to describe the practice of psychological medicine. He was a German doctor and used the word 'Psychiatrie' in 1808.

Semple DM *et al.*, eds. *Oxford Handbook of Psychiatry*, 1st edn. Oxford University Press, 2005, p. 20.

59. B. Thomas Szasz has expressed strong views against the current conceptual models of disease in psychiatry. Antipsychiatry refers to a heterogeneous school that challenges the fundamental theories and practices of psychiatry. Aubrey Lewis was an English psychiatrist associated with the Maudsley Hospital. Adolf Meyer proposed psychobiology.

Johnstone EC *et al.*, eds. *Companion to Psychiatric Studies*, 7th edn. Churchill Livingstone, 2004, p. 4 Table 1.2.

60. D. Interpretation is an interview technique and not a boundary violation. It is increasingly realized that subtle violations of doctor–patient boundaries often occur in psychiatric setting. Boundary crossing is defined as intentional or unintentional incursions occurring during a therapeutic relationship. When such boundary crossings produce harm to the patient, then they are called boundary violations. This can be both sexual and non-sexual violation.

Kay J and Tasman A, eds. *Essentials of Psychiatry*. Wiley, 2006, p. 65, Table 5.5.

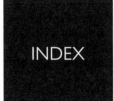

INDEX

Key: ■ denotes question, ■ denotes answer